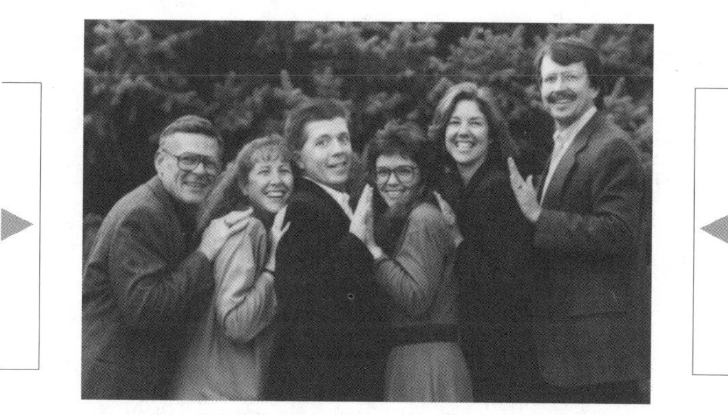

Our "Compacted" Compact Clinicals Team

Dear Valued Customer,

WELCOME to Compact Clinicals. We are committed to bringing mental health professionals up-to-date diagnostic and treatment information in a compact, timesaving, and easy-to-read format. Our line of books provides current, thorough reviews of assessment and treatment strategies for mental disorders.

We've "compacted" complete information for diagnosing each disorder and comparing how different theoretical orientations approach treatment. Our books use nonacademic language, real-world examples, and well-defined terminology.

Enjoy this and other timesaving books from Compact Clinicals.

Sincerely,

Melanie Dean, Ph.D.
President

Compact Clinicals Line of Books

Compact Clinicals currently offers these condensed reviews for professionals:

For Physicians

Bipolar Disorder: Treatment and Management

Trisha Suppes, M.D., Ph.D. & Paul E. Keck, Jr., M.D.

For Clinicians

Attention Deficit Hyperactivity Disorder

The latest assessment and treatment strategies

C. Keith Conners, Ph.D.

Bipolar Disorder

The latest assessment and treatment strategies

Trisha Suppes M.D., Ph.D. and Ellen Dennehy, Ph.D.

Borderline Personality Disorder

The latest assessment and treatment strategies

Melanie Dean, Ph.D.

Conduct Disorders

The latest assessment and treatment strategies

J. Mark Eddy, Ph.D.

Depression in Adults

The latest assessment and treatment strategies

Anton Tolman, Ph.D.

Obsessive Compulsive Disorder

The latest assessment and treatment strategies

Gail Steketee, Ph.D. and Teresa Pigot, M.D.

Post Traumatic Stress Disorder

The latest assessment and treatment strategies

Matthew J. Friedman, M.D., Ph.D.

Depression in Adults

The latest assessment and treatment strategies

Third Edition

Anton Tolman, Ph.D.

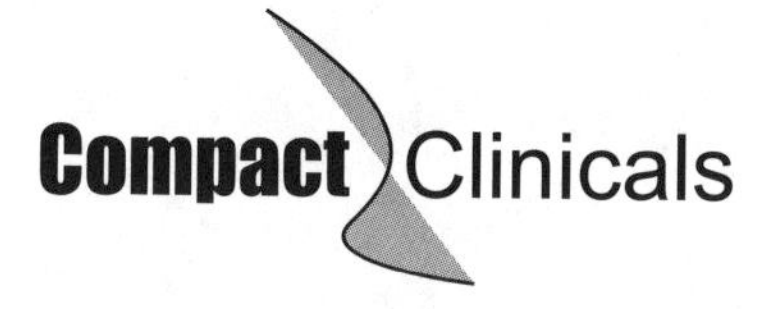

This book is intended for use by properly trained and licensed mental health professionals, who already possess a solid education in psychological theory, research, and treatment. This book is in no way intended to replace or supplement such training and education, nor is it to be used as the sole basis for any decision regarding treatment. It is merely intended to be used by such trained and educated professionals as a review and resource guide when considering how to best treat a person with major depressive disorder.

Depression in Adults

The latest assessment and treatment strategies

Third Edition

by

Anton Tolman, Ph.D.

Compact Clinicals

Published by: Compact Clinicals
7205 NW Waukomis Dr., Suite A
Kansas City, MO 64151
816-587-0044

Copy Editing: In Credible English, Inc.®
P.O. Box 1309
Sandy, UT 84091

Book Design: Coleridge Design, Kansas City, Missouri

Library of Congress Cataloging in Publication data:

Tolman, Anton O.
Depression in adults : the latest assessment and treatment strategies / by Anton Tolman.—3rd ed.
p. ; cm.
Includes bibliographical references and index.
ISBN 1-887537-24-4
1. Depression, Mental. 2. Depression, Mental–Treatment. I. Title.
RC537.T647 2005
616.85'2706–dc22
2004028250

10 9 8 7 6 5 4 3 2 1

Read Me First

As a mental health professional, often the information you need can only be obtained after countless hours of reading or library research. If your schedule precludes this time commitment, Compact Clinicals is the answer.

Our books are practitioner oriented with easy-to-read treatment descriptions and examples. Compact Clinicals books are written in a nonacademic style. Our books are formatted to make the first reading, as well as ongoing reference, quick and easy. You will find:

- ***Anecdotes*** — Each chapter contains a fictionalized account that personalizes the disorder entitled, "From the Patient's Perspective."
- ***Sidebars*** — Narrow columns on the outside of each page highlight important information, preview upcoming sections or concepts, and define terms used in the text.
- ***Definitions*** — Terms are defined in the sidebars where they originally appear in the text and in an alphabetical glossary on pages 73 through 76.
- ***References*** — Numbered references appear in the text following information from that source. Full references appear on pages 85 through 96.
- ***Case Examples*** — Our examples illustrate typical client comments or conversational exchanges that help clarify different treatment approaches. Identifying information in the examples (e.g., the individual's real name, profession, age, and/or location) has been changed to protect the confidentiality of those clients discussed in case examples.
- ***Key Concepts*** — At the end of each chapter, we include a review list of key concepts from that chapter. Use these lists for ongoing quick reference as well as for reviewing what you learned from reading the chapter.

Contents

Chapter One:
General Information about Depression

This chapter answers the following:

- **How Common is Major Depression?** —This section describes the number of people with the disorder and how the rate of depression has increased in recent years.
- **What Causes Depression?** —This section outlines recent research supporting an integrated explanation for what causes depression, including psychological, environmental, and biological factors.
- **What is the Likelihood of Recovery?** —This section discusses recurrence rates and severity as well as the correlation between mortality and depression.

DEPRESSION occurs so frequently in the population that it has been called the "common cold of psychopathology."[1, 2] It is a serious emotional disorder that can range in intensity from mild to severe and is estimated to be one of the world's leading causes of disability.[3] In an historic document that addressed the nation's mental health for the first time, the U.S. Surgeon General noted that, in a given year, approximately seven percent of the U.S. population suffers from a mood disorder. Depression is the largest contributor to these mood disorders, according to the Surgeon General.[4] Clearly, depression is a serious, global public health concern.

In this book, the term "depression" refers exclusively to the clinical condition, Major Depressive Disorder, as defined in the ***Diagnostic and Statistical Manual, 4th Edition, Text Revision [DSM-IV (TR)].***[5]

Mild depressive symptoms include:

- Sadness
- Loss of interest in life's activities or pleasures
- Low self-esteem
- Changes in sleeping and eating patterns
- Poor attention and concentration
- A negative outlook on the future

People with mild depression can usually continue work and handle their responsibilities, but function below their normal level. Severe depressive episodes often present additional symptoms of slowed thought and movement, prominent thoughts of guilt, suicidal thoughts and/or plans, and psychotic symptoms (impaired awareness of reality).

Depression is characterized by a persistent disruption in mood with simultaneous interruptions in the person's thoughts, behaviors, and physiological functioning. To be diagnosed, the disorder must disrupt social functioning in major areas of life (e.g., work, school, family/marital).

> *This Compact Clinicals book summarizes some of the latest information on:*
> - *Prevalence, cause, and likelihood of recovery (this chapter)*
> - *Diagnosing the disorder (chapter two)*
> - *Diagnosing and treating suicide risk (chapter three)*
> - *Psychological treatments (chapter four)*
> - *Biological treatments (chapter five)*

learned helplessness — passive behavior based on the expectation that one's efforts will fail

rumination — thinking the same thoughts repeatedly

> *One recent study concluded that genetic risk factors for depression may be stronger in women than in men.*[15]

How Common is Major Depression?

Studies show major depression to be very common, but prevalence is difficult to establish. Results of two, large-scale, well-designed studies on the prevalence of depression found that between five and 15 percent of Americans suffer from major depression at any given time. Similarly, six to 17 percent of Americans will suffer from a major depressive episode at some point in their lifetime.[6, 7]

The course of the disorder does not appear to vary by gender (and there is no difference in prevalence of the disorder in pre-pubescent males and females).[7, 8, 9] However, prevalence studies consistently indicate higher rates of depression among women, which does not appear to be due to the different methods used in the studies.[10] Interestingly, Martin Seligman, Ph.D (reknown researcher and author on depression-related topics) believes that women are more depressed than men because women:[8]

- Are more prone than men to develop *learned helplessness* due to social factors.[7]
- Tend to engage in more *rumination* and negative thought patterns, which can increase or amplify depression.[9, 11]
- Equate standards of beauty and acceptance with images seen in the media. Women who fit the standard set forth in the media represent a small percentage of the population. In women, this pressure creates overall dissatisfaction with their bodies, decreases self-esteem, and increases guilt.[12, 13]

Women may experience depression more often due to greater levels of chronic life stress, low sense of mastery over their environment, and more ruminative coping styles.[14] Other reasons why women may experience depression more often than men include having less economic power, experiencing emotional stressors more intensely, suffering higher rates of sexual and physical abuse, undergoing hormonal changes, or suffering from hypothyroidism (a metabolic disorder that mimics depression).[4, 14]

From The Patient's Perspective

Finally went to a therapist today. Pat Owen. I guess it's time again; I just seem to be getting worse; can't get up and going. Feels like that black hole again; how I hate that black hole. I'm scared that this time I won't be able to get out of it. It seems hopeless. Dad keeps needing more and more since Mom died. Can't seem to pull myself together to help him. I feel so out of shape, and I need some sleep.

Rates of depression in the U.S. and other western-hemisphere countries appear to be increasing. Early studies demonstrate as much as a 10:1 increase in the rate of depression over the course of the century.[8, 16–18] Further, a recent study indicates that psychological factors, such as: self-disparagement, feeling worthless, and having trouble concentrating, are more specific and stronger predictors of future depression than more "medical" symptoms, such as insomnia.[19]

As of the 2000 U.S. Census, approximately 28.7 million women (about 20 percent) and 16.5 million men (about 12 percent of men) will suffer from depression in the course of their lifetime; however, mental health professionals will treat only about 11 percent of these individuals.

What Causes Depression?

The common question, "Is depression due to a chemical imbalance or psychological processes?" reflects the typical distinction made between emotional/mental processes and physical processes. To lessen the social stigma of a "mental" disorder, medical, psychiatric, and other professional groups have historically promoted the concept of depression and other mental disorders as "diseases." Unfortunately, this promotes the belief that depression is a simple condition with a simple solution. Nothing could be further from the truth.

Chapters four and five address theories about depression's causes from either a psychosocial or a biological perspective, making it easier to understand the origins of specific treatment methods that evolved from those theories.

In fact, mental/emotional functioning and physiology are intertwined and affected by ongoing social relationships and environmental events. Studies indicate that learning changes brain structure, indicating a complex interaction between brain structure, brain chemistry, and environmental/social events.

The emerging model of depression is highly interactive, emphasizing that onset is not a "one-way street," but that risk factors constantly interact to shape one's chances of becoming depressed. This model emphasizes the principle of *equifinality* and the ongoing interaction between genes, environment, internal thought patterns, and social factors that combine in unique ways and cause depression.[20] This "interactive" model is based on evidence that while genes may increase a person's sensitivity to stress, they may also shape personality factors (such as the tendency to seek out situations that make one sad or to engage in bad relationships) that actually **increase** the person's chance of depression.[21, 22] Further, studies with both animals and humans suggest that expression of genetic vulnerabilities is heavily determined by interactions with the early parenting patterns and environmental situations.[23, 24] A recent review of the impact of heredity, parenting behavior, and environmental situations (such as the neighborhood in which the family lives), shows that all interact to shape children's behavior and personality.[24]

equifinality — the theory that there may be many different pathways that lead to a similar clinical outcome (e.g., schizophrenia, depression, and autism)

Although genetic factors may make one person more prone to depression than another, environmental events might interact with genes, shaping the way they affect brain function, making the brain more sensitive to new stress. Similarly, modeling and parental behaviors as well as the behaviors of others (e.g., peers, husband, wife) may shape the development of thought patterns (such as pessimism) and behaviors (such as shyness) that may make depression more likely to occur.

A recent summary of the integrative model of depression emphasizes the relationships among these elements that interact to cause depression:[25]

- **Biological or genetic vulnerability** — These involve multiple genes that interact with environmental influences, shape the nature of a person's brain chemistry, and may shape personality characteristics like emotional instability.[26, 27] *Neurotransmitters* (brain chemicals), such as *serotonin* and *norepinephrine,* help regulate mood and are closely connected to the human stress-response system.[26]
- **Psychological vulnerability** — Involves behaviors shaped by factors such as shyness and seeking excessive reassurance.[28] Recent studies indicate that solving problems protects people from stressful life events — while avoidance strategies can cause depression.[29]
- **Stressful Life Events** — Stressful life events, especially personal loss or physical or sexual abuse, appear to increase the likelihood of depression by making the brain's stress response system more hypersensitive and overwhelmed.[27]
- **Unique Stress Reactions** — Research clearly indicates the potential for stress reactions to result in substantial changes in brain neurochemistry and structure, including development of a "persistently hypersensitive stress-response system."[30] Early trauma may damage or decrease neuron growth in the *hippocampus*, an important brain structure linked with mood disorders.
- **Cognitive Factors** — A person's general thoughts and beliefs about the world and relationships may cause depression (e.g., those who generally have a pessimistic view of the world are more prone to depression than those who are optimistic).
- **Interpersonal Effects and Social Demands** — Social and emotional factors that affect relationship quality are related to stress; positive social support reduces this stress while negative relationships increase it.

Key mediators of depression include loneliness and difficulty maintaining positive self-esteem.[31, 32] Factors such as loneliness may form the "bridge" to depression. For example, neglected or abused children with genetic vulnerability to depression may develop shyness because they believe others think they are stupid or unlovable. Such children may also develop a pessimistic

neurotransmitters — chemical agents in the brain that affect behavior, mood, and feelings

serotonin — a neurotransmitter from the indoleamine group, which affects central nervous system functioning and appears to moderate the effects of many other neurotransmitters

norepinephrine — type of catecholamine that affects central nervous system functioning

hippocampus — an important part of the limbic system involved in working memory and other functions

When a child experiences a severe stress, such as losing a parent, the emotional trauma may increase the brain's sensitivity to stress and vulnerability for depression.

There is evidence that being viewed negatively by a close friend or loved one can trigger depressive relapse.[33]

outlook on life and believe their situations will not change. This leads to social behaviors that cause others to reject them, confirming their world view and leaving them feeling isolated and lonely. This may trigger a depressive episode.

One year following diagnosis of depression, 40 percent of individuals still have symptoms severe enough to maintain the diagnosis; 20 percent have some continued symptoms but no longer meet depression diagnostic criteria; and 40 percent have no mood disorder. Some of these cases, especially those with mild depression, subside without treatment.[5]

A person's first depressive episode may occur during young adulthood — a crucial time for developing and stabilizing interpersonal relationships and learning to cope effectively with stress.[35, 36]

What is the Likelihood of Recovery?

Depression, once thought to be mostly a single-episode acute disorder, is now considered a chronic disorder that occurs in multiple episodes with periods of remission and relapse (similar to asthma, diabetes, or arthritis). This new understanding alters traditional strategies for treatment and relapse prevention.[34] Factors that seem to predict a relapse include:

- **A prior history of depressive episodes** — Thought patterns, interpersonal relationships, and neurochemical changes in the brain (resulting from the first depressive episode) impact subsequent episodes.[36] The chance of recurrent depressive episodes increases with each episode experienced; relapse rates are 50 to 85 percent for those experiencing a single episode, 70 percent for those with two prior episodes, and 90 percent for those with three prior episodes.[2, 37] A severe first episode increases the risk of relapse as well.
- **The presence of chronic physical disorders and/or other psychiatric disorders** — Most instances of lifelong, recurrent depression co-occur with other psychiatric disorders, often anxiety. These *comorbid* types of depression tend to be more persistent and severe than depression that occurs without other psychiatric disorders.[38]
- **Elapsed time between recovery and the next episode** — With each recurring episode, this time decreases.
- **Ineffective diagnosis and treatment** — Studies indicate that half of the clients who recover from depression initially did **not** receive preventative treatment in the month prior to relapse.[38] Some indicate that less than half of depressed clients are properly diagnosed, and that less than half of those treated achieve remission.[19, 26]

comorbid — the simultaneous presence of two or more disorders

Probably the most serious complication of depression is suicide (including unsuccessful attempts). Estimated suicide completion rates are as high as 15 percent among depressed people, a rate that is three to four times higher than in other psychiatric disorders and 36 times higher than the general population.[39]

Chapter three covers suicide assessment and treatment recommendations in detail.

Depression has other widespread health effects:

- Increased death rate for those over 55 (non-suicidal)
- "Markedly increased likelihood of death" among elderly admitted to nursing homes within one year[5]
- Immune system inhibition[1]
- Link to chronic pain (in part, because of shared neurotransmitter systems affected during depression)
- Increased risk of cardiac disease and likelihood of death following cardiac events[40–42]

Although the exact mechanisms by which depression may influence response to a heart attack are unknown, depression can trigger increased nervous system activation, disrupt heart rhythms, thicken blood, and increase inflammation.

Key Concepts for Chapter One:

1. Overall, six to 17 percent of Americans suffer a major depressive episode at some time in their lives.
2. Roughly 20 percent of women and 11 percent of men in the U.S. will suffer from depression.
3. Those with depression typically suffer from a persistent disruption in mood with simultaneous interruptions in thoughts, behaviors, and physiological as well as social functioning.
4. Diagnosis requires significant impairment in major areas of life (e.g., employment, academic, family/marital).
5. Depression is considered a chronic disorder that occurs in multiple episodes with periods of remission and relapse (similar to asthma, diabetes, or arthritis).
6. Integrated models of depression's cause focus on the intertwining of genetics, environmental and social factors, stress, and internal thought patterns.
7. Estimated completed suicide rates among depressed persons are as high as 15 percent.
8. Depression can inhibit the immune system, relate to chronic pain, be linked to heart disease, and predict death following cardiac events.

Chapter Two: Diagnosing Depression

This chapter answers the following:

- **What Criteria Are Used to Diagnose Major Depression?** —This section presents DSM-IV (TR) criteria as well as diagnostic clarifiers and challenges.
- **What Are Typical Characteristics of Those With Depression?** —This section describes typical presentations of "withdrawn" and "agitated" depression.
- **What Other Depression Types and Classifications Exist?** —This section covers atypical depression, melancholia, dysthymia, and seasonal affective disorder.
- **What Tools Are Available for Clinical Assessment of Depression?** —This section provides general guidance for clinical interviewing as well as assessment tools and laboratory findings.
- **What Differentiates Depression from Other Disorders?** —This section addresses differential diagnosis issues for bipolar disorders, primary medical conditions, dementia, dysthymia, and schizoaffective disorder.

DIAGNOSING depression presents a variety of challenges because the disorder can present quite differently from client to client and has so many impacting social, physiological, and psychological factors. In addition, the clinician must carefully differentiate depression from a number of other medical and psychiatric disorders with similar symptoms.

What Criteria Are Used to Diagnose Major Depression?

The DSM-IV lists the criteria (figure 2.1, shown on the next page) for diagnosing a depressive episode. These criteria are reprinted with permission of American Psychiatric Association, Diagnostic and Statistical Manual of Mental Disorders, Fourth Edition, Text Revision, Washington, D.C., American Psychiatric Association, 2000.[5]

Diagnostic Clarifiers

The DSM-IV label, "Major Depressive Disorder," actually defines a group or family of related forms of depression. The first decision a clinician needs to make in diagnosis is whether or not the current episode is the patient's first and only episode. If this is the case, the situation requires the diagnosis of Major Depressive Disorder, Single Episode. Patients suffering more than one instance of depression (indicated by at least two months with no symptoms of depression), would be diagnosed as having Recurrent Depression.

mood incongruent — the content of the delusion (or hallucination) does not match the depression

hallucination — sensory perceptions without external stimulation; hearing voices or seeing things others do not; a compelling perceptual experience of seeing, hearing, or smelling something that is not actually present

mixed episode — a mixture of symptoms indicating both mania and depression

psychotic — impairment in awareness of reality, including symptoms of delusions and/or hallucinations

Figure 2.1
DSM-IV Criteria for Major Depressive Disorder[5]

A. Five (or more) of the following symptoms have been present during the same 2-week period and represent a change from previous functioning; at least one of the symptoms is either (1) depressed mood or (2) loss of interest or pleasure.

Note: Do not include symptoms that are clearly due to a general medical condition, or *mood-incongruent* delusions or *hallucinations.*

1. depressed mood most of the day, nearly every day, as indicated by either subjective report (e.g., feels sad or empty) or observation made by others (e.g., appears tearful).

Note: In children and adolescents, can be irritable mood.

2. markedly diminished interest or pleasure in all, or almost all, activities most of the day, nearly every day (as indicated by either subjective account or observation made by others).
3. significant weight loss when not dieting or weight gain (e.g., a change of more than 5 percent of body weight in a month), or decrease or increase in appetite nearly every day.

Note: In children, consider failure to make expected weight gains.

4. insomnia or hypersomnia nearly every day.
5. psychomotor agitation or retardation nearly every day (observable by others, not merely subjective feelings of restlessness or being slowed down).
6. fatigue or loss of energy nearly every day.
7. feelings of worthlessness or excessive or inappropriate guilt (which may be delusional) nearly every day (not merely self-reproach or guilt about being sick).
8. diminished ability to think or concentrate, or indecisiveness, nearly every day (either by subjective account or as observed by others).
9. recurrent thoughts of death (not just fear of dying), recurrent suicidal ideation without a specific plan, or a suicide attempt or a specific plan for committing suicide.

B. The symptoms do not meet criteria for a *Mixed Episode*

C. The symptoms cause clinically significant distress or impairment in social, occupational, or other important areas of functioning.

D. The symptoms are not due to the direct physiological effects of a substance (e.g., a drug of abuse, a medication) or a general medical condition (e.g., hypothyroidism).

E. The symptoms are not better accounted for by bereavement, i.e., after the loss of a loved one; the symptoms persist for longer than two months or are characterized by marked functional impairment, morbid preoccupation with worthlessness, suicidal ideation, *psychotic* symptoms, or psychomotor retardation."

Reprinted with permission of American Psychiatric Association, *Diagnostic and Statistical Manual of Mental Disorders, Fourth Edition, Text Revision,* Washington, D.C., American Psychiatric Association, 2000.[5]

Detailed Specifiers

DSM-IV explicitly endorses a number of more detailed specifiers for current depressive episodes. These specifiers enable clinicians to further define the nature and estimate the future course of the disorder. They include:

- Descriptors of course, such as "chronic" (continuous symptoms of depression for two years or more) or "recurrent" (more than one episode of depression); if the depression is recurrent, the clinician could indicate how well the person recovered between episodes of depression (called inter-episode recovery), and whether or not there is a seasonal pattern (e.g., onset and remission at characteristic times of the year; usually beginning in fall or winter and remitting in spring)
- Prominent features of the disorder, such as:
  - **Catatonic** — a rare condition usually involving symptoms like lack of speech, aimless moving about, or total absence of movement and unresponsiveness
  - **Melancholic** — worse depression in the morning; awakening early
  - **Atypical** — mood brightens at times, excessive sleeping, heavy feeling in arms/legs
- Onset of the disorder, such as **postpartum** (beginning within four weeks of child birth)

Double Depression

According to the DSM-IV, approximately 20 to 25 percent of individuals diagnosed with major depression, whether a single episode or recurrent, suffer from so-called "*Double Depression,*" in which both *dysthymia* and major depression are present. Both disorders should be diagnosed since each provides significant implications for treatment and prognosis.

double depression — intense depressive episode that is superimposed on the milder, chronic depressive disorder called dysthymia

dysthymia — a persistent, low-level depression that has been ongoing for two years or more

Depression Severity

Clinicians rate the depression severity based on the number of symptoms manifested by the patient and the degree of impact on daily functioning. At one end of the spectrum, those with a minimum of five diagnostic symptoms receive a "mild" rating (as long as the clinician considers functional impairment to be "minor"). Clinicians use severe ratings when patients present more than five symptoms and when the degree of impairment "markedly interferes" with functioning.[5] There are also categories for rating the depression in partial or full *remission* (absence of symptoms) as well as a final "unspecified" category.

remission — absence of all symptoms; full remission if there have been no symptoms for at least six months, partial remission if no symptoms for less than six months

When rating someone's depression as "severe," the clinician must specify whether psychotic symptoms of delusions (false beliefs) and/or hallucinations (e.g., sensory disturbances such as hearing voices) are present. If psychotic features are present, the clinician needs to specify whether those features are *mood congruent*. When diagnosing "Depression with Psychotic Features," the psychotic features must have developed after or concurrently with the depressive features.

mood congruent — the content of the delusion or hallucination matches depressive symptoms

Recurrent Depression

The clinician must carefully review the client's previous depression history, which helps ensure accurate diagnosis, assists in treatment and prognosis determinations, and targets the need for relapse prevention. For example, clients experiencing their second major depressive episode may warrant the expanded diagnosis of "Recurrent Depression."

The modifier "recurrent" can be significant because it affects estimates of client prognosis (see chapter one, page 5).

Other Diagnostic Challenges

DSM-IV attempts to narrow complex information related to biological, social, and psychological functioning into specific symptom criteria for major depression, making it necessary to be aware of several diagnostic factors:[43]

- **The prototype approach to diagnosis**, which requires only a number of specific symptoms to be present to make a diagnosis. This can result in a variety of disorders being classed as "depression."
- **DSM-IV omits some well-researched symptoms of depression**, such as hopelessness and social withdrawal.
- **DSM-IV does not effectively differentiate between depression and grief** (the only diagnostic difference being the death of the loved one).
- **Some disorders classified as "adjustment" disorders** seem to have more in common with depression but present fewer symptoms.

DSM-IV has at least 15 types and subtypes of mood disorders leading to over 50 diagnostic code combinations.

From The Patient's Perspective

Saw Owen today. She wants me to have a complete physical with blood tests. I don't know when I'm going to have time to do that. I know there is nothing physically wrong with me, except that I have gained a lot of weight recently. Dad needs me to take him to the dentist; I feel guilty both for taking time off work and for not being there more for Dad. At least I should take him to the dentist since I can't seem to help him in any other way. Terry needs me, too. I don't think I've been much of a spouse lately. I wish they would all just leave me alone.

What are Typical Characteristics of Those with Depression?

Depending on the duration, severity, and symptoms (e.g., anxiety or psychotic symptoms) of their depression, client presentations may vary widely. Of these, episode length and severity are the most important factors, being directly proportional to the presentation of the typical symptoms listed below. Clients with "mild" depression vary the most in their initial presentation; those with "moderate" to "severe" depression vary less. The following sections describe typical presentations for "withdrawn" depression and less-common, "agitated" depression.

These general statements about presentation help clinicians recognize overt symptoms of depression; individual clients will fluctuate in how well they fit these generalized examples.

Typical Presentation — "Withdrawn" Depression

Many depressed clients manifest feelings (affect), thoughts (cognitions), and behaviors consistent with being sad or withdrawn, such as:

- **Affect** — Depressed clients' emotional display or "affect" may be either *constricted* or *labile*. Clients who are experiencing acute suicidal thinking (see chapter three) often appear very tense with tight facial expressions and noticeable tension in their hands, face, or shoulders.
- **Cognitions** — Depressed clients often manifest a pessimistic thought pattern, discounting positive life events and criticizing their own behaviors, decisions, or actions. Clients may express helpless, powerless, or hopeless feelings. *Aaron Beck* and his colleagues describe a typical cognitive triad in the depressed client that involves:[44]
  1. **A negative view of the self**, typically expressed as statements about being defective, deprived, or inadequate. This view may extend to blaming the self as a source of pain to others (e.g., "Everyone would be happier if I were dead.").
  2. **The tendency to interpret external events as negative** despite plausible alternative explanations (e.g., "The store clerk could see how stupid and slow I am," versus "The store clerk was grumpy with me because he was having a bad day.").
  3. **A pattern of viewing the future as negative** and predicting future failures and disasters (e.g., "I will never be happy in my marriage; I can't get better.").
- **Behaviors** — Depressed clients are often withdrawn and quiet. Voice tone is soft, making them difficult to hear. They frequently hang their head, avoid eye contact, and can appear socially isolated. They may not volunteer information about themselves and may frequently respond by saying, "I don't know."

constricted — appearing apathetic and not displaying much emotion

labile — marked and rapid mood shifts (e.g., a client may smile briefly when asked about past hobbies, then burst suddenly into tears)

Aaron Beck — a psychiatrist prominently known for his cognitive-behavioral theory and treatments for various mental disorders

Those with depression often move slowly, as if they are very tired or in pain, and they may appear indecisive or unwilling to make decisions.

Typical Presentation — "Agitated" Depression

A withdrawn client is more likely to complain of a lack of appetite and of sleeping more than usual. However, an "agitated" client may report overeating, even in the absence of appetite.

middle insomnia — waking in the middle of the night, often unable to gradually return to sleep

terminal insomnia — waking early and not being able to get back to sleep (e.g., at 4:00 or 5:00 a.m.)

In contrast to the more "withdrawn" forms of depression, clients with "agitated" depression may often appear angry with themselves or with others.

Clients may be more concerned with how others treat them rather than expressing self-criticism, although themes of self-criticism may also be present.

Clients with "agitated" depression tend to show small differences in presentation when compared to clients experiencing "withdrawn" depression. These differences may show up in the client's report rather than be clearly visible. An "agitated" client may experience slightly more **rumination**, which disrupts sleep onset, and may report higher rates of *middle insomnia* as well as *terminal insomnia*.

Those with "agitated" depression manifest affect, cognitions, and behaviors, such as:

- **Affect** — Clients with "agitated" depression often appear preoccupied rather than withdrawn and generally tense with either a constricted or labile affect. They may express resentment more often than guilt, although both are often present. They may also look as if they feel hurt inside and do not know how to express it.
- **Cognitions** — While clients with agitated depression may still manifest thoughts associated with Beck's Cognitive Triad, their thought patterns focus on feeling slighted, ignored, or rejected. They interpret events around them negatively with an emphasis on how unfair life can be. They also describe high expectations for others as well as themselves and feel hurt or resentful when these expectations are not met. Finally, they may see the future as bleak and actively hostile to their goals.
- **Behaviors** — The most obvious behavior that may be associated with "agitated" depression is increased motor movement. Even while remaining seated, they may frequently move their head, arms, or legs. There may be occasional bursts of anger directed toward the clinician (e.g., "I thought I came here for you to give me answers, not for me to answer questions.") These brief outbursts may be followed by contrition or self-blame. They may spontaneously volunteer information about themselves, but can appear impatient with the interview.

Suicide Assessment

Because of the high degree of association between depression and suicidal ideation and behavior, clinicians working with depressed patients should routinely screen and evaluate clients for suicide potential.

Data suggests that precise predictions of suicide rates are often unreliable. Therefore, clinicians should focus on assessing the risk level of suicide rather than trying to specifically predict whether or not a patient will be suicidal. This allows the clinician to help manage and lower the risk in a given individual.[45, 46]

Chapter three covers suicide assessment and treatment in detail and includes: a clinical decision model for assessing suicide potential, various diagnostic tools, key issues in managing suicide risk, and treatment interventions.

What Other Depression Types and Classifications Exist?

As previously noted, depression consists of a "family" of related conditions; common subtypes and distinctive classifications include atypical depression, melancholia, dysthymia, and seasonal affective disorder (SAD).[43]

Atypical Depression

DSM-IV permits the diagnosis of depression with "atypical features" if the core criteria are met and the following symptom groups exist:

- **Mood brightens** in response to actual or potential positive events
- **Two** of the following exist:
  - Significant weight gain/increase in appetite
  - Hypersomnia
  - Leaden paralysis (heavy feeling in arms or legs)
  - Long-standing interpersonal sensitivity that results in significant impairment
- **Symptoms do not meet** criteria for catatonic or melancholic features

Atypical depression was initially thought to represent a type of "chronic over-reactive dysphoria" and hypersensitivity to disappointment in relationships.

Melancholia

Long described as "endogenous," this subtype of depression indicates a more biologically based disorder that occurs independent of stressful life events. While some research supports these assumptions, DSM criteria for melancholic depression have typically changed with each manual edition, leading to some ongoing confusion about describing the disorder.

The latest edition, DSM-IV (TR), permits classification of a depressive episode with "melancholic features" including:

- **Either** the loss of pleasure in all or almost all activities **or** the lack of reactivity to usually pleasurable stimuli (does not feel much better even temporarily when something good happens)
- **Plus three or more** of the following symptoms:
  - The depressed mood is experienced as distinctly different from the kind of feeling experienced after the death of a loved one.
  - Depression is regularly worse in the morning.
  - The person awakens early in the morning — at least two hours before usual awakening time (terminal insomnia).

- The person displays marked psychomotor agitation or retardation.
- The person suffers from significant anorexia or weight loss.
- The person experiences excessive or inappropriate guilt.

Dysthymia

Many individuals with dysthymia may develop major depression at some point in their life.

Less understood than depression, dysthymia may often emerge in childhood or adolescence, and thus is often seen as becoming an integrated part of a person's personality development. As a result, those suffering from this long-term, chronic condition tend to have a very pessimistic outlook on life and poor social skills. Treatment implications revolve around helping clients develop a new sense of themselves rather than just returning to a "normal" state. Because clients come to regard the mood disturbance as their "normal" level of functioning, they are often surprised when the clinician informs them that continued treatment can resolve their dysthymia. In addition, dysthymia tends to respond poorly to medication treatment and tends toward a long-term course even in psychotherapy.

Dysthymia sufferers may present depressive symptoms, but they are often capable of demonstrating a much greater amount of positive emotion than those with depression. For example, they may become tearful, but still respond to humor or smile appropriately.

Diagnostic criteria for dysthymia include:

- The person suffers a depressed mood for most of the day, for more days than not, for at least two years (with the absence of symptoms occurring for no more than two months).
- The presence of **two or more** of the following symptoms while depressed:
  - Poor appetite or overeating
  - Insomnia or hypersomnia
  - Low energy or fatigue
  - Low self-esteem
  - Poor concentration or difficulty making decisions
  - Feelings of hopelessness

It is possible for an individual to suffer from a major depressive episode superimposed upon an existing dysthymic disorder, resulting in the so-called, "Double Depression."

While dysthymia responds well to normal treatments for depression, the course of therapy is often slightly longer, particularly if the dysthymia has lasted for several years (especially since adolescence).

However, in cases where both disorders may be present, the clinician would not diagnose dysthymia unless it had been present before the onset of the depressive episode. If the patient initially experienced depression, the clinician would not diagnose dysthymia unless there had been a full remission of depression (two months of normal mood) prior to onset of the dysthymia.

Seasonal Affective Disorder (SAD)

For the past two decades, the concept that climatic elements could influence a form of depression has been growing in influence. The essential concept behind SAD is that seasonal fluctuations in available sunlight may trigger underlying problems with the person's *circadian rhythms*. Problems with the concept have emerged, however, including the following:

circadian rhythms — the daily regulation of sleep-wake cycles and activity patterns

- Seasonal fluctuations may exist in non-depressed as well as in depressed populations.
- There is no elevated prevalence of SAD within sufferer's families, suggesting no genetic foundation for the disorder.
- There is considerable overlap in symptoms between SAD and other types of depression.
- There is a lack of significant evidence for a differential treatment response (early studies showed that phototherapy or light therapy brought some improvement to persons with non-seasonal depression).
- Individuals with SAD may respond to some traditional antidepressants such as Monoamine Oxidase Inhibitors (MAOI).

DSM-IV permits classification of SAD as a "seasonal pattern" in recurrent depression; however, it is relatively difficult to meet the conditions for this situation:

This criteria is only met if the seasonal variation is not due to a psychosocial stressor, such as scheduled unemployment, return to school, etc.

- A regular, temporal relationship exists between the onset of a major depressive recurrence and a particular time of the year (e.g., the person consistently becomes depressed during the fall or winter or, more rarely, the summer).
- Full remissions also occur at a characteristic time of the year (e.g., the person's depression always disappears when spring begins).
- The most recent two years must demonstrate the seasonal pattern of depression, and there has not been any period of time when the season came and went without depression.
- Over the course of the person's lifetime (not just the past two years) the seasonal nature of the depression has to "substantially outnumber" any non-seasonal episodes of depression.

What Tools are Available for Clinical Assessment of Depression?

Diagnosing and assessing depression involves gathering specific information from clinical interviews, self-report instruments, structured interviews, and psychometric assessment instruments.

This section presents an overview of diagnostic tools; detailed information on assessment instruments appears in ***Appendix: Depression Assessment Instruments****.*

Clinical Interviewing

During the clinical interview, clinicians need to gather information about medical history, family history, and social functioning.

The following medical disorders can cause symptoms of depression:

- ***Thyroid disorder** often mimics depression (but is also accompanied by dry skin, hair loss, and sensitivity to cold temperatures).*
- ***Diabetic conditions** can produce mood swings, depression, irritability, and fatigue.*
- ***Anemia** can produce fatigue, sluggishness, and depression.*
- ***Cancer** (some forms can produce depression).*
- ***Pre-Menstrual Dysphoric Disorder** (formerly Pre-Menstrual Syndrome) also may cause depressive symptoms.*

Medical History — Because many medical disorders can mimic or cause depression, the clinician can only diagnose major depression if the symptoms are not due to a general medical condition.

There are a number of problematic issues that clinicians evaluating clients who present both with possible depression and a history of medical illness must consider. These include:[47]

- Possible overlap between the vegetative symptoms of an illness and depression, including fatigue, lack of appetite, and other disturbances of sleeping and eating (e.g., sleep apnea that results in excessive fatigue and sleep disturbance), including substance abuse, addiction, or symptoms of withdrawal (e.g., for alcohol, cocaine, methamphetamines, or marijuana). Young male patients who present with depression should also be screened for inhalant abuse.
- Some illnesses produce pain and disability, which could be confused with depressive symptoms.
- Depressed mood may directly result from diagnosis of a life-threatening condition or a chronic disorder, which could lead to major life changes and affect body functioning.
- Some medications or other medical treatments (e.g., chemotherapy, beta-blockers, steroids, estrogen, sedatives, and others) can produce symptoms that appear to be depressive symptoms.

For a summary of medical conditions thought of as causally related to depression, refer to Stevens and colleagues.[47]

Practically speaking, these issues make the clinician liable for finding out the date of the client's last medical exam and screening for the possibility of current medical conditions and treatments.

In situations where medical conditions are present, the clinician should work with or consult with the physician to determine how the illness and/or treatments might affect depression. Clinician and physician may then discuss approaches to psychotherapy and medical care that maintain the client's physical health while reducing depression symptoms.

Individual and Family Psychiatric History — To help confirm the diagnosis and shape the treatment plan, include questions regarding:

- Recurrent depressive episodes
- Severity of initial episode
- Severity of current episode
- Any previous suicide attempts or thoughts

- Previous psychiatric hospitalization
- Significant stressors (such as childhood abuse, death of a parent, parental divorce)
- Evidence of personality disorder

Because genetics also influence whether or not a person may become depressed, assessment and initial screening of clients presenting for treatment should always include an examination of family psychiatric history, including family history of suicide.

Studies have indicated that depression occurs 1.5 to 3 times as frequently in first-degree relatives of a depressed individual as in the general population.[5]

Social Functioning History — Collecting a social and occupational history will help identify any impairment in functioning required to diagnose major depression. Ask about school or job performance, socializing, status of friendships, and status of intimate relationships.

Self-Report Instruments and Structured Interviews

The most commonly used instruments for helping assess depression fall into four classes: self-report instruments, structured interviews, combined instruments, and psychometric instruments.

Figure 2.2, on the following page, lists these instruments by category; chapter three details suicide assessment instruments. The appendix offers more detailed information on each instrument as well.

Physiological Laboratory Findings

Lab findings, although helpful in continued research regarding the cause or effects of depression on human physiology, do not appear to add precision to diagnostic decisions at this time.

A recent review of potential diagnostic laboratory tests concluded that origins and biology of depression are more complex than was originally thought.[48] Reviewers noted that, in the past decade, no laboratory "gold standard" has emerged for diagnosing depression. Tests previously thought promising, such as tests of metabolites of brain neurotransmitters or the well-known Dexamethasone Suppression Test, have largely proven unreliable. Sleep studies need further research but may promise clinical utility in predicting treatment response and monitoring outcome of treatment interventions. Brain imaging techniques, such as CT Scans, may help with differential diagnosis in cases of physiological disorders that mimic apparent depression. However these techniques are still costly and probably should not be considered for routine diagnostic use.

Laboratory tests used to detect abnormalities include:

- *Sleep and waking EEGs*
- *Measures of neurotransmitter levels or their metabolites in blood*
- *Cerebrospinal fluid, urine, or platelet receptor functioning*
- *Dexamethasone Suppression Test*
- *Functional and structural brain imaging*
- *Neuroendocrine challenges*
- *Evoked potentials*

Figure 2.2 Depression Assessment Instruments

Type	Use	Instruments Available*
Self-report instruments	Self-report instruments are used to either screen for depression in various settings or to classify subjects for research purposes. They are generally checklists or inventories that are completed by the client.	• Beck Cognitive Checklist (CCL) • Beck Depression Inventory - 2 (BDI-2) • Center for Epidemiological Studies Depression Scale (CES-D) • Cornell Scale for Depression in Dementia (CSDD) • Geriatric Depression Scale (GDS) • Zung Self-Rating Depression Scale (SDS)
Structured interviews	Structured interviews are instruments in which trained clinicians follow a strict interview format that probes for possible symptoms of psychopathology. In some cases, the clinician may be interviewing others (e.g., the Cornell Scale for depression in Dementia); in other cases (e.g., the Diagnostic Interview Schedule or the Composite International Diagnostic Interview), the instrument was explicitly designed so that lay persons could administer the interview.	• Composite International Diagnostic Interview (CIDI) • Diagnostic Interview Schedule (DIS) • Hamilton Rating Scale for Depression (HRSD, sometimes called HAM-D) • Schedule for Affective Disorders and Schizophrenia (SADS) • Structured Clinical Interview for DSM-IV Axis I Disorders (SCID)
Combined instruments	Combined instruments are those that have a self-report component completed by the client, followed by a semi-structured interview completed by the mental health professional.	• Harvard Department of Psychiatry/National Depression Screening Day scale (HANDS) • Prime-MD
Psychometric instruments	Psychometric assessments are used to facilitate diagnosis and describe personality characteristics.	• Minnesota Multiphasic Personality Inventory (MMPI) • Rorschach Inkblot Test • Thematic Apperception Test (TAT)

*For more information on each of these instruments, refer to the appendix on pages 77–83.

What Differentiates Depression from Other Disorders?

Clinicians must differentiate between depression and:

- *Bipolar Disorder*
- *A Primary Medical Condition*
- *Substance-Induced Mood Disorders*
- *Dementia*
- *Dysthymia*
- *Schizoaffective Disorders*

When diagnosing major depression, the clinician must rule out the possibility that the client's symptoms are related to another medical or psychiatric condition.

Bipolar Disorders

Clinicians must rule out any previous or current history of mania in a client with depressive symptoms, since depression-specific treatments can sometimes precipitate a manic episode. For example, in a client with a history of mania, lithium has usually been considered the treatment of choice. If a clinician unknowingly administered antidepressant medication instead to this person, it could trigger a manic episode. Since those who are manic frequently engage in harmful or destructive behavior toward themselves or others, this is an important differential diagnosis.

Mania is characterized as either a manic episode, mixed episode, or *hypomanic* episode. DSM-IV defines a manic episode as an "abnormally and persistently elevated, expansive, or irritable mood."[5 (p. 328)] Mania often manifests in little need for sleep, excessive energy, and impulsive, irrational, and destructive behavior. Clinicians can screen for mania by asking if the patient has ever experienced times when they didn't need much sleep and yet felt invigorated or energized.

hypomanic — exhibiting symptoms of mild mania

There is a strong link between depressive episodes and mania. According to the DSM-IV, there is a five to 10 percent likelihood that a person having their first depressive episode will later experience a manic episode.[5] Since there is typically no previous history of mania at the time of presentation, clinicians cannot immediately distinguish these individuals from the population of persons suffering only depression. In these cases, the differential diagnosis can only be made over time.

Primary Medical Condition

The clinician needs to determine if depressive symptoms might be related to or caused by a primary medical condition. This differentiation is important for medical professionals to ensure adequate and specific treatment and for non-medical professionals to make appropriate referrals and coordinate care. Between eight and 10 percent of all depression cases are directly related to a primary medical condition.[49, 50] For example, many clinicians see patients with depression symptoms that result more from sleep apnea or other sleep disorders.

Clinicians should always consider the onset of symptoms and the presence of a known physical disorder as well as laboratory results and family history.

DSM-IV lists these medical concerns as being related to mood disturbance:[5]

- Degenerative neurological conditions (e.g., Parkinson's disease, Huntington's disease)
- Cerebrovascular disease (e.g., stroke)
- Metabolic conditions (e.g., vitamin B1 deficiency)
- Endocrine conditions (e.g., hyper- and hypo-thyroidism, hyper- and hypo-parathyroidism, hyper- and hypo-adrenocorticism)
- Autoimmune conditions (e.g., systemic lupus, erythematosus)
- Viral or other infections [e.g., hepatitis, mononucleosis, human immunodeficiency virus (HIV)]
- Certain cancers (e.g., carcinoma of the pancreas)

Substance-Induced Mood Disorder

Differentiating between a primary mood disorder and a substance-induced disorder can be difficult at times given the high propensity with which depressed individuals self-medicate with alcohol or street drugs.

The diagnosis of a substance-induced mood disorder, new to DSM-IV, involves a disturbance of mood judged by the clinician to be directly related to the physiological effect of a substance (e.g., street drugs, medication, or toxin exposures). For this diagnosis to be made in relation to street drugs, there must be evidence of intoxication, withdrawal, or both. For example, cocaine withdrawal may produce depressive symptoms.

The DSM-IV notes that symptoms persisting more than four weeks may indicate mood-related disturbances, rather than substance withdrawal, as substance withdrawal symptoms usually last four weeks or less. DSM-IV also clarifies that some legitimate medications prescribed for other conditions or reasons (e.g., alpha-methyldopa for hypertension or birth-control pills) can either produce depressive symptoms or can exacerbate the course of a preexisting depressive disorder.

Differentiate substance-induced mood disorder by carefully considering:

- Date of onset (which condition came first?)
- Drug abuse/dependence history
- Severity of symptoms compared with those expected from intoxication or withdrawal from specific substances
- Prior history of depressive episodes

Dementia

dementia — loss of intellectual capacity in such areas as memory, judgment, and reasoning, usually due to brain deterioration

A client with a strong family history of dementia and no personal or family history of depression should be much more prone to dementia. However, a client with a history of multiple depressive episodes and long-lived and well-functioning relatives would have a greater likelihood of being depressed.

Determining whether elderly individuals suffer from depression or *dementia* can be difficult because many depressed patients in geriatric settings appear demented (and many of the staff may assume this is the case). Cognitive impairment in these instances is referred to as "pseudo-dementia." Differentiation of these conditions requires clinicians to obtain a good medical history, paying particular attention to personal and family history of dementia, cancer, stroke, high blood pressure (which can produce strokes or other forms of brain damage), diabetes, and other medical conditions that could damage brain tissue.

The clinician should carefully evaluate these functional deficits to determine whether or not the person's inhibited abilities stem from brain damage or depression. For example:

- **Memory Loss** — It is not unusual for depressed elderly patients to display "short-term" memory loss while retaining long-term memory. This short-term loss actually is due to the distractibility or concentration difficulty inherent in cases of depression. Usually dementia affects long-term memory as well as verbal or visual memory.

- **Sleep** — Sleep disturbance is common for both dementia and depression. With depression, the sleep disturbance involves insomnia (often a result of rumination) or excessive sleeping. With dementia, sleep disturbance can result from being confused about when and where to sleep.
- **Appetite** — Changes in appetite are common with both depression and dementia. With depression, clients are usually aware of their diminished or increased appetite and will acknowledge this change. With dementia, the client usually displays little awareness of this change.
- **Grooming or Hygiene Skills** — With both depression and dementia, these behaviors decrease. However, with depression, poorer grooming skills are related to a loss of motivation rather than a loss of skill. With dementia, people begin to lose their ability to perform such grooming behaviors as brushing teeth or combing hair. To differentiate between the two during an assessment, the clinician can ask the client to demonstrate "how" to do certain grooming behaviors.

The clinician should also consider the acuteness of onset. With dementia, there is typically a gradual deterioration or a step-wise loss of functions (associated with vascular dementia). With depression, onset is often abrupt in a person with a good pre-illness history. As with all other differential diagnoses, useful data can come from reviewing family history and previous history of depression.

Schizoaffective Disorder

In cases of severe depression, psychotic symptoms may be present and may dominate the client's initial presentation. These symptoms may include confused speech, comments about hearing voices, or expressed beliefs that appear to be unfounded (i.e., delusions). These symptoms may obscure an underlying depression.

The difference between a depressive disorder with psychotic features and schizoaffective disorder is that in the latter, psychotic symptoms must occur for at least two weeks without the presence of the depressive symptoms. Additionally, in order to diagnose schizoaffective disorder, depressive symptoms must be present more than half of the duration of the illness. If the mood disturbance meets criteria for adult major depression and is relatively brief compared to the length of the psychotic symptoms, then schizophrenia and major depressive disorder are diagnosed separately.

Key Concepts for Chapter Two:

1. Diagnostic criteria for major depression include a number of clarifiers related to the course of the disorder, its prominent features, and the onset of symptoms.
2. Those with "withdrawn" depression typically present a constricted or labile affect, a pessimistic thought pattern, and quiet and withdrawn behaviors.
3. Those with "agitated" depression typically appear more preoccupied than withdrawn, demonstrate more motor movement and sometimes frequent verbal outbursts, express resentment more often than guilt, and look as if they're unsure how to express hurt feelings.
4. Depression types also include atypical depression, melancholia, dysthymia, and seasonal affective disorder (SAD).
5. Thyroid disorder, diabetic conditions, anemia, some forms of cancer, and pre-menstrual dysphoric disorder (formerly pre-menstrual syndrome) can all produce symptoms similar to depression, making medical history a critical part of diagnosis.
6. In addition to a medical history, family psychiatric history (especially because of the genetic component in depression) and social functioning are important areas of assessment.
7. A number of self-report instruments, clinical interviewing tools, combined instruments, and psychometric instruments exist for diagnosing depression.
8. Differential diagnosis must address the possibility that the patient's symptoms are not characteristic of bipolar disorder, a primary medical condition, substance-induced mood disorders, dementia, dysthymia, or schizoaffective disorders.

Chapter Three:
Managing Suicide Risk in Depressed Patients

This chapter answers the following:

- **How Do I Assess the Risk Factors Associated with Suicidal Patients?** — This section presents key predictors of suicide risk and diagnostic tools available for measuring that risk.
- **What Interventions Can Be Used with Suicidal Patients?** — This section discusses issues surrounding hospitalization vs. outpatient treatment as well as psychological and biological treatment strategies.
- **What Key Issues Impact Treatment Strategies?** — This section covers issues related to treatment environments and legal concerns.

IN 2000, suicide was the 11th leading cause of death in the United States; it was the third leading cause of death among persons 15–24 years old.[51] It is the most frequently encountered emergency by mental health professionals.[45]

The statistics are sobering — for those with major depression, suicidal thinking is common; about 15 percent of those diagnosed with major depression eventually commit suicide; and many who kill themselves see medical professionals prior to taking their lives.[45] As a result, everyone working with depressed patients should be aware of suicide risk factors, possible interventions, and legal and treatment considerations.

White males commit 73 percent of suicides, with older, white males having the highest incidence rates. An older, white male who mentions suicide should be taken very seriously.[52, 53]

With an average of 10 percent of the population depressed at any one time, 4,000,000 people could be contemplating suicide at any moment. Compare this to the .01 percent of the general population (approximately 30,000 people) that commits suicide each year (based on information provided by the National Center for Health Statistics). The purpose of risk assessment is to help the clinician decide in which group the patient most likely belongs.

How Do I Assess the Risk Factors Associated with Suicidal Patients?

Because research has been inconclusive on the effectiveness of instruments for **predicting** suicidality among depressed patients, clinicians should turn their diagnostic attention to assessing the relative risk of suicide, which is greatest for those who have attempted suicide before.[45] First-time suicide attempters are most often disturbed by acute mental disorders (Axis I on the DSM), while more chronic forms of suicidality tend to be associated with personality disorders (Axis II on the DSM).[45]

The therapeutic goal of risk management is to reduce the chance that the patient will attempt suicide.

Once clinicians have assessed suicide risk level, the risk must be managed to reduce the crisis. Figure 3.1, on the following page, illustrates the overall approach for managing suicide risk.

Figure 3.1 Managing Suicide Risk

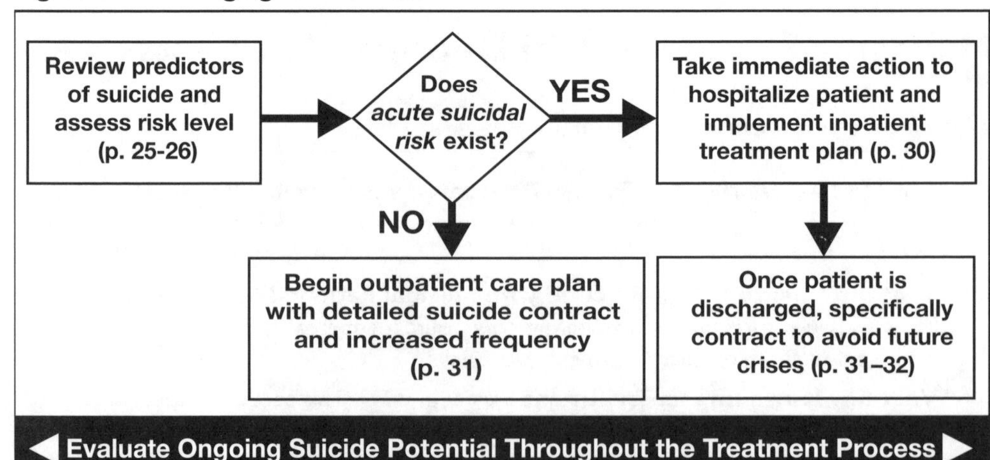

acute suicidal risk — possible suicidal behavior within hours

The following sections detail how to:

- Evaluate the overall level of suicide risk
- Talk with patients about suicide
- Use diagnostic instruments to assess risk

Evaluating the Level of Suicide Risk

Figure 3.2, on pages 25 through 26, integrates information from clinical history, observations, results from a mental status interview, information from the patient's significant others, data from psychological instruments, and suicide risk estimators to rate overall level of suicide risk. These risk factors must be evaluated in terms of their relationship to one another for any given patient.[54] The success of using such a complex decision model appears to depend much on the evaluator's skill, experience, and familiarity with interacting risk factors.[45]

Evaluate the patient's suicide plans in terms of:

- **How detailed is the plan?** — The more detailed, the **higher** the risk.
- **What is the *lethality* of the method contemplated?** — The more lethal, the **higher** the risk.
- **How available are the means to implement the plan?** — The more available, the **higher** the risk.
- **How near are mitigating or helping resources?** — The greater the support system of friends and family members, the **lower** the risk.
- **What is the patient's level of self-control?** — The poorer the impulse control, the **higher** the risk.
- **Has the patient attempted suicide in the past?** — Previous suicide attempts **increase** risk.

lethality — the probability of a fatal outcome, measured as the elapsed time between the use of the method and death plus the likelihood that medical intervention will not prevent death

Figure 3.2 Overall Level of Risk: Intensity of Factors

<table>
<tr><th>Key Risk Factors[54]</th><th>Mild</th><th>Moderate</th><th>Severe</th><th>Extreme</th></tr>
<tr><td>Resolved Plans and Preparations
• Having specific suicidal thoughts
• Level of planning (amount of detail, securing of resources, rehearsal)
• Lethality of method</td><td>• Claiming lack of reasons for living and/or wishing to die
• Thinking about suicide
• Wanting or expecting to make an attempt
• Lack of deterrents to making an attempt
• Talking about death or suicide</td><td colspan="2">• Having the courage/sense of competence to attempt suicide
• Availability of a means to carry out a suicide plan
• Frequently thinking about suicide; intensity of thoughts
• Planning suicide elements (e.g., location, time, method, impact upon others)
• Alarming behaviors indicating intention to die (e.g., giving away possessions, saying good-bye)</td><td>• Increased preoccupation with plan details
• Evidence of scheduling time for planning or carrying out a plan
• Rehearsal of plan elements or experimental action
• Access to firearms and other highly lethal methods
• Previous attempt with highly lethal methods</td></tr>
<tr><td>Negative Life Stressors/ Events[55]
Negative life events are related to the severity of suicidal symptoms in non- or first-time attempters, but not for multiple attempters.[55]</td><td>• Employment problems (e.g., being unemployed, having an inconsistent work history)[56]
• Feelings of worthlessness, shame, guilt, legal problems, loss of close relationships, and chronic overwork
• Chronic sleep problems</td><td colspan="3">• Having experienced recent personal loss death, divorce
• Experiencing life stressors at a level where suicide is a consideration (including chronic pain or medical symptoms) TERMINAL CA OR A.I.D.S (Full Blown)
• Having acute psychiatric symptoms (e.g., severe depression, psychosis, intense anxiety)</td></tr>
<tr><td>Co-occurring Disorders
Multiple medical and/or psychological problems increase suicide risk.[45]</td><td>• Presence of anxiety disorders or substance abuse
• Presence of cancer, epilepsy, arthritis, or other chronic, often-painful illnesses</td><td colspan="3">• Presence of anxiety disorders or substance abuse, as well as chronic, painful physical illnesses, along with sense of hopelessness[57]
• Presence of hopelessness and helplessness</td></tr>
<tr><td>Previous Suicide Attempts
— At least one prior suicide attempt (more likely due to personality factors)</td><td>No other risk factors</td><td>ANY other significant findings (e.g., suicidal desire or ideation, resolved plans</td><td>Two or more risk factors</td><td>Severe or extreme symptoms from the resolved plans and preparations domain</td></tr>
<tr><td>No Previous Suicide Attempts
— First suicidal crisis or no history of suicide attempts (more likely due to acute illness)</td><td>Limited or mild suicidality (vague thoughts, no specific plan)</td><td>Moderate-to-severe symptoms, especially resolved plans</td><td>Moderate-to-severe findings related to resolved plans and preparations AND at least one other risk factor</td><td>Severe or extreme symptoms related to resolved plans and preparations AND two or more other risk factors</td></tr>
</table>

Figure 3.2 (continued) Overall Level of Risk: Intensity of Factors

Key Risk Factors[54]	Mild	Moderate	Severe	Extreme
Family History	• Family history of depression or suicide • Chaotic family of origin background (e.g., parental divorce or death, mental health problems, frequent moves, substance use) • History of physical or sexual abuse	Family history predictors (listed in "mild" risk column at left) combined with: • Previous suicide attempts • Suicidal thinking • Having other acute clinical symptoms Suicide rates are highest among divorced and widowed.[45, 58]		
Impulsive Behavior	History of impulsive behaviors (e.g., changing jobs without considering impact, quickly formed relationships, spending sprees) and suicidal thinking		History of mild-to-moderate impulsive behaviors and evidence of suicidal **planning** (see page 25)	
Support Systems • Positive social support • Self control • Problem-solving abilities • Ability to write about feelings and thoughts	Lack of support systems or problems with support systems (e.g., isolates self)	Symptoms of suicide planning (see page 25) despite presence of some support systems		Symptoms of suicide planning (see page 25) and little or no presence of support systems
Alcoholism/ Drug Abuse	About 18 percent of all alcoholics eventually kill themselves. The relationship to suicide risk may be through disruption in social supports that results from substance abuse.			
Personality Factors	Those who are generally ruminative and/or anxious	Persons who are highly anxious, feel panicked or lonely, or are emotionally unstable (e.g., borderline)	• Those who are angry in addition to being depressed; have a history of violence toward themselves or others • Younger people who may harbor a desire for "murderous revenge" (they may tend to commit suicide as a way of "punishing" those they are angry with)	

Talking with Patients about Suicide

Ask clear, simple questions about whether or not the patient wants to die and if they have a plan for committing suicide. The goal is to determine how emotionally upset or unstable the person is, how likely the person is to act on their suicidal ideation, and how difficult it would be to rescue the person if they were to use the method they are considering. Utilize an "ascending approach" for the patient interview, beginning with questions about nonspecific suicidal thinking, then moving into a review of specific passive and active suicidal thoughts.[59]

Alone, any factor may be insufficient to produce suicidal behavior. Patients tend to manifest several of these factors at once or over time, even over their lifetimes. Be aware of long-term patterns and interactions between specific factors when assessing suicide risk.

Nonspecific suicidal thinking involves questions like:

- "Have you ever thought of hurting yourself?"
- "Have you had suicidal thoughts recently?"

Reviewing specific passive suicidal thoughts might involve asking questions like:

- "Do you **want** to commit suicide?"
- "Might you do so sometime if things get worse?"
- "Do you think about suicide but have no specific plans?"
- "Do you sometimes wish you could die?"

Reviewing specific active suicidal thoughts might involve asking:

- "When are you planning to commit suicide?"
- "How would you do that? What method are you planning to use?"
- "Where do you think about killing yourself?"

From The Patient's Perspective

I am starting therapy with Owen, and I sure hope it helps. She asked me questions about whether or not I had ever thought about killing myself. I guess I have thought about it quite a bit lately; I even wondered if I could find the combination to my dad's gun safe. I've never been this down before that I really thought about a plan for committing suicide. Somehow, I think this should scare me a little more than it does. Maybe there's some pill I can take to make these thoughts go away? Sometimes, I think my family would like it better if I weren't around; but other times, I think they'd really be hurt.

Patients who have made use of more lethal methods in the past tend to be more:

- *Serious about actually dying*
- *Disappointed that they did not succeed with previous attempts*
- *Likely to use highly lethal methods in future attempts*

The clinician then asks for a description of all methods the patient has used in the past and evaluates how much time and effort the patient has expended in considering current suicide plans. This information is vital because the patient is likely to repeat past behaviors. Certain methods of attempting suicide are much more lethal or dangerous than others; for example, attempting suicide by shooting oneself is much more likely to result in death than attempting an overdose.

Similarly, if a person has a history of prior attempts, it is very important to understand why they did not die. For example, if the person wakes up and calls for help, it indicates some desire to live. On the other hand, if the only reason the person did not die was that they pulled the gun's trigger too hard and the bullet did not strike a critical area, such a patient should be considered a much higher risk.

The presence of multiple attempts, especially of low lethality, is likely to indicate the presence of a personality disorder, as compared with an acute clinical disorder. Capturing a solid clinical history of prior attempts is directly relevant to developing an effective treatment plan for reducing depression and the risk for future suicide.

Using Diagnostic Instruments to Assess Suicide Risk

Figure 3.3 on page 29 provides a brief overview of these tools with additional detail provided in the appendix.

A number of diagnostic instruments exist for evaluating suicide risk. No suicide risk estimator or instrument has been proven effective for predicting all suicide risk. These instruments evaluate specific aspects of risk but should be integrated with information from other sources.

Figure 3.3 Tools for Evaluating Suicide Risk

Tool Name	Info Measured/Collected	Appropriate Age for Use	Remarks
Beck Hopelessness Scale (BHS) [60, 61]	Pessimism	17 years+	Good complementary tool
Beck Scale for Suicidal Ideation[30, 60, 62]	Severity of suicidal ideation	Adolescents and adults	Best for monitoring quality and quantity of changes in suicidal thoughts
Scale for Suicidal Ideation (SSI)[63]	Elevated suicidal risk that bears closer monitoring	17 years+*	Must be used by a trained clinician
Suicidal Intent Scale (SIS)[64]	Suicidal preparations, planning, circumstances of a prior attempt, and the reactions to prior attempt (e.g., disappointment)	For adults, (may be effective with adolescents)	Used typically with SSI
Firestone Assessment of Self-destructive Thoughts[46]	Suicide risk	16 years+	Administered in a group setting
Suicide Probability Scale (SPS)[60, 65]	Attitudes and behaviors relevant to suicide risk; concepts relevant to suicide rather than specific risk factors	14 years+	Self-report scale
Los Angeles Suicide Prevention Center Scale**[66]	Risk for callers on a crisis line or drop-in to prevention center	15–adult	Determines patient management strategies
Adult Suicide Ideation Questionnaire (ASIQ)[67]	Specific suicidal thoughts and behaviors; frequency within past month	18 years+	Self-report scale
Suicidal Behavior History Form (SBHF)[68]	Information on a patient's history of suicidal behavior	Adults/ adolescents	Evaluates and documents previous suicidal behaviors.
Risk-Rescue Rating Scale*[69]	Current or prior suicide attempts or plan risk and method lethality	No specific age; studied in those 10+ years	Measures level of suicide attempt risk and likelihood of rescue given methods being considered
Lethality of Suicide Attempt Rating Scale (LSARS)*[70]	How lethal previous suicide attempts have been and potential lethality of future attempts	No specific age	
Reasons for Living Inventory[71]	Patient beliefs that could mediate suicidal behaviors	Adults	Discriminates between suicidal and non-suicidal patients; both 48- and 72-item versions available

* Has been used with adolescents from age 13

** Found in the appendices of *The Suicidal Patient: Clinical and Legal Standards of Care, 2nd Edition.*[45]

What Interventions can be used with Suicidal Patients?

One of the most widely cited works on standards of care for suicidal patients is Bruce Bongar's classic work, ***The Suicidal Patient.***[45]

Although there are no definitive signs or measures that predict who will commit suicide, clinicians should pay special attention to those risk factors that have been associated with previous suicide attempts, ongoing use of alcohol or drugs, hopelessness, and degree of interpersonal conflict (which may also be related to potential homicidal ideation).[45]

Because it is very difficult to accurately **predict** completed suicide, focus instead on selecting **the best strategy to effectively manage or lower the suicide risk**. Management first involves reviewing the specific predictors of suicide (see pages 25 through 26) and assessing whether or not the risk is acute (requiring hospitalization). Then, the clinician can develop a treatment strategy based on inpatient or outpatient considerations, the patient's history as a non- or single-attempter vs. a multiple-attempter, and what combination of psychological and biological treatments may be warranted. Once a clinician has determined that a patient is suicidal, the first key treatment issue is whether or not the patient should be hospitalized.

Managing Inpatient Care Issues

After making a decision to hospitalize, the clinician needs to ensure that the person evaluating the crisis has sufficient evidence for making such a decision. For example, a patient who is angry or does not want to be hospitalized may convince police officers or mental health workers (depending on state law) that there is a misunderstanding, and they do not want to kill themselves. This could result in a suicidal patient being released.

Reduce the ongoing potential for suicide after the initial suicidal crisis by:[72]

- *Including the family in treatment*
- *Realistically informing the patient about probable treatment length and effectiveness as well as his/her expected role*
- ***Regularly*** *questioning the patient about suicidal feelings, intent, and plans (including possible repeated use of a suicide risk instrument)*

The clinician should ensure that any "gatekeeping" evaluator understands the patient's history, suicidal symptoms and plans, and the risk factors that led to the referral. In addition, the clinician should be sure that the hospital can provide the level of restraint necessary to ensure the patient's safety. In most cases, the clinician will be expected to provide hospital staff with specific patient information identifying the need for inpatient hospital care after intake. Additionally, the clinician needs to maintain contact with the hospital treating staff about discharge planning for the patient. Once the patient is discharged, the clinician can develop an outpatient treatment plan, featuring:

- An explicit plan for future suicidal crises, which includes: regular reviews of suicidal ideation, intent, plan, and status of risk factors as well as patient and family involvement.
- Increased session frequency and/or scheduled, between-visit contacts (e.g., via phone)
- Steps for removing potential suicide instruments, perhaps with help from family or friends
- Regular evaluation of the patient's willingness to emotionally engage in the treatment relationship and responsiveness to treatment
- (For the clinician), professional consultations (and documented results) with a colleague experienced in patient management

The clinician may be able to contact a family member or friend to have guns (or medications) taken away/locked up. In this case, the suicidal individual will not ***necessarily*** *find another method.*[58]

Using Suicide Contracts

A common suicide intervention for clinicians, prior to hospitalization, is to specifically contract with the patient to not commit suicide. This is a fairly common procedure when clinicians believe the risk may be minimal or chronic in nature. Contracts are usually a verbal or written agreement between the clinician and patient that the person will not commit suicide without using the emergency plan developed or without first speaking with the clinician.

Although the use of so-called "no-harm contracts" is controversial, overall, many studies find that most individuals, both professionals and lay persons, are positive about the use of such agreements.[73, 74]

Use these contracts with caution because:

- Some patients think the contract means that they should contact their clinician **only** when they are acutely suicidal and desperate.
- Others may have a strong need to be compliant and reasonable and may sign a contract despite serious misgivings about living up to it — precipitating a crisis due to feelings of guilt and shame.
- Clinicians might gain a false sense of security from such a contract.

More explicit contracts appear more useful than general contracts with suicidal patients because they ask patients to:[74]

As a clinical (rather than legal) tool, these contracts may provide information about the patient's level of suicidal intent and their sense of control.

- Agree with specific therapeutic treatment goals, including to "live a long life with more pleasure and less unhappiness than I have now"
- Learn better ways to manage their emotions
- Specifically name contact and backup persons with phone numbers
- Work with their clinician
- "Openly renegotiate" the contract when it expires

In contrast, general contracts require the patient to sign a statement that, for a specific time, they would speak with a friend or relative if feeling suicidal. Some contracts add a basic promise to call a crisis line if the patient stopped taking medications, seriously thought about committing suicide, or took any action towards planning suicide.[74]

Using Psychological Treatment Strategies for Suicidal Patients

Until the crisis is over and the patient is no longer intensely suicidal, psychotherapy should focus on increasing the patient's sense of choices available to them and their sense of being emotionally supported. Key strategies include:

- Reducing psychiatric symptom intensity (e.g., instilling a sense of hope, decreasing vegetative symptoms, teaching methods to cope with anxiety and frustration, etc.)

- Teaching problem-solving methods to cope with major life stressors, such as divorce or unemployment

Chapter four details cognitive-behavioral approaches to treatment.

These strategies are consistent with a recent study pointing out that, while there is a need for more research on treatment effectiveness for suicidal patients, cognitive-behavioral approaches that emphasize a problem-solving focus seem to reduce suicidal behavior for most persons studied, at least for short-term interventions.[75] The data from multiple attempters in this study suggests that longer-term treatment may be needed to address underlying personality disorders and to develop personal skills for accessing resources and coping with life crises.

For first-time attempters, once the immediate suicidal crisis is past, the best way to reduce potential attempts is to immediately try to reduce the symptoms or mitigate the life event producing the crisis. For multiple attempters, this strategy's value may be limited. More intensive follow-up of longer duration should focus on reducing what precipitated the immediate crisis and on achieving longer-term ability to prevent future crises.[57]

Family members need to understand the factors that indicate suicide risk and ways to ensure safety (e.g., hospitalization).

Involving family members or other concerned parties in evaluating and responding to suicide risk can be advantageous.[76] They typically provide increased social support for the distressed patient, valuable information for evaluating ongoing risk, and backup safety options should the suicide risk increase between clinical contacts.

Using Biological Treatment Strategies for Suicidal Patients

psychotropic medications — medications that affect behavior, emotions, and/or cognitive processes

Suicidal patients may respond positively to medications. (See chapter five for the theory and use of *psychotropic medications* in treating depression.) However, clinicians should be aware that many of these medications may take a number of days to work; thus, for patients at imminent risk, this may not be a safe course to consider. In addition, significant numbers of patients commit suicide using preventive medications, which is less of a risk with the newer antidepressants.

Refer to chapter five for more specific information on ECT.

Whether administered on an inpatient or outpatient basis, Electroconvulsive Therapy (ECT) may be an appropriate consideration for patients who express suicidal ideation AND one of the following symptoms:

psychotic depression — severe depression that includes delusions (false beliefs) or hallucinations (perceptual distortions such as hearing voices or seeing things that are not there)

- Refuse to eat
- Experience *psychotic depression*
- Are at high risk for suicide and have not responded well to other treatments

What Key Issues Impact Treatment Strategies?

Treating suicidal patients often involves dealing with issues outside those of typical treatment environments, including:

- **Dealing with Insurance Restrictions/Limitations** — Managed care and similar organizations may restrict patient care even during a suicidal crisis. Although this situation is being slowly addressed via court cases (e.g., Andrews-Clarke v. Travelers), clinicians may need to talk with patients about coverage restrictions and advocate on a patient's behalf to appeal these decisions.[77]

  In addition, clinicians need to be familiar with their state's laws and procedures for involuntarily committing a suicidal patient to a facility, considering the patient's insurance benefits and the willingness to be voluntarily hospitalized. Hospital choice also may hinge on whether or not the patient has insurance.

- **Using Confidentiality Waivers** — Suicidal patients need to know that confidentiality may be waived to protect their safety and that the clinician will take their suicidal thoughts and comments seriously.
- **Developing an Emergency Plan** — Develop an emergency plan for outpatients who display suicidal or even homicidal behaviors. Discuss this plan with the patient early in the first session, providing a written procedure to follow in an emergency.
- **Recognizing Countertransference Issues** — *Countertransference* often occurs when the clinician reacts to the patient with their own sense of helplessness, worries about being able to handle a suicidal crisis, and fear of potential legal outcomes. This reaction is magnified by the suicidal person's negative experiences of telling others about their thoughts, making them leery of sharing this information with the clinician because they expect the same reaction. Clinicians who present themselves as competent, calm, and able to take action may help resolve the crisis and calm the patient.
- **Handling Legal Concerns** — Because of the litigation potential surrounding suicide cases, clinicians need to practice in a way that is both ethical and legally defensible. In malpractice or negligence cases, courts and juries tend to evaluate the situation in terms of how "reasonable" the clinician's actions were in comparison to those of "average," prudent clinicians of similar training and experience.[45]

Once hospitalized (whether voluntarily or not), clinicians should be involved in the facility's ongoing treatment and discharge planning.

Clinicians who wish to know more about the potential legal ramifications of a specific waiver should consult an attorney.

Although emergency plans vary widely, they often include elements, such as: calling 911, contacting the clinician after hours through a phone service or on-call line, or making use of community-based crisis hotlines.

countertransference — patient issues that trigger feelings in the clinician, such as anxiety, a sense of helplessness, feeling out of control, or feelings that may "echo" the patient's own feelings

Courts do not expect clinicians to have perfect judgment and accept that predicting suicide can be an almost impossible task.[45, 78]

To mitigate the risk of liability:

- Provide high-quality patient care, focusing on the patient's health and well-being.
- Document specific findings regarding the patient's degree of risk, the clinician's reasoning during the crisis, and decisions made.
- Consult with other professionals and document these consultations, particularly when making a decision to manage a suicidal patient on an outpatient basis.
- Follow prudent standards for decision-making and developing adequate documentation.

Key Concepts for Chapter Three:

1. The risk of suicide is greatest for those who have attempted suicide in the past.
2. Evaluating suicide risk requires analyzing the detail level of the plan, the lethality of the method contemplated, the accessibility of the means to implement the plan, the nearness of mitigating resources, the patient's level of self-control, and the existence of a previous suicide attempt.
3. Other key suicide risk factors can involve family history, impulsive behaviors, alcoholism/drug abuse, angry or vengeful personality factors, negative life stressors/events, and co-occurring disorders (such as anxiety disorders and chronic, painful medical disorders).
4. Although a number of suicide risk assessment tools exist, no one tool has proven effective in predicting suicide attempts. Clinicians must balance these tools with information from other sources.
5. Inpatient care issues for suicidal patients involve clear communication between clinician and hospital, oversight of discharge planning, and development of an explicit plan for preventing future suicide crisis once the patient has been discharged from the hospital.
6. Outpatient care typically involves use of a suicide contract that the patient signs, agreeing to talk to someone when feeling suicidal.
7. Cognitive-behavioral psychotherapy that focuses on problem solving has reduced short-term suicidal behavior for most persons studied.
8. Family members should be involved in treating a suicidal patient to help ensure increased social support, evaluate ongoing risk, and provide backup safety options should the suicide risk increase between clinical contacts.
9. For those at high risk for suicide, especially those experiencing psychotic depression, electroconvulsive therapy (ECT) may prove effective.
10. Key issues in treatment planning include insurance restrictions/limitations, confidentiality waivers, emergency planning, countertransference, and legal concerns.

Chapter Four: Psychological Treatments for Depression

This chapter answers the following:

- **What is the Psychodynamic Approach for Treating Depression?** — This section highlights two perspectives: classical psychodynamic thought and object relations.
- **What is the Interpersonal Therapy (IPT) Approach for Treating Depression?** — This section describes the interpersonal therapy approach as well as treatment strategies and effectiveness.
- **What is the Behavioral Therapy Approach for Treating Depression?** — This section describes the behavioral therapy approach as well as treatment strategies and effectiveness.
- **What is the Cognitive-Behavioral Approach for Treating Depression?** — This section describes the cognitive behavioral therapy approach as well as treatment strategies and effectiveness.
- **How Does Group Therapy Help Those Suffering from Depression?** — This section covers theory, treatment, and outcome for two major forms of group therapy; cognitive behavioral and interactional /psychodynamic group therapy.

INTEGRATED models of depression's origins emphasize the interactions between environmental and biological factors. This chapter focuses on psychosocial and environmental elements that theoretically contribute to major depressive disorder and individual treatments associated with each of these approaches:

- **Psychodynamic** — The psychodynamic approach assumes that historical events and the developmental aspects of personality interact to cause a patient's current psychological problems. Some researchers indicate that life experiences are the most statistically important influence on depression scores.[80]
- **Interpersonal** — The interpersonal therapy (IPT) approach is a modern, short-term, psychodynamic therapy that supports an active role for the clinician and addresses depressive symptoms in relation to current events and relationships.
- **Behavioral** — The behavioral approach focuses on how people's behaviors, specifically social skills, impact their ability to receive *positive reinforcement* from their environment. Since reinforcement increases the measurable frequency of behavior, a person's inability to receive *reinforcement* for healthy behavior directly affects depressive symptoms.
- **Cognitive Behavioral** — Cognitive behavioral theories focus on how the person's internal thoughts, images, and belief systems affect their behavior. While there are several different cognitive theories, treatment methods tend to incorporate behavioral strategies because of the interplay between cognitions and behavior.

In a recent survey, 36 percent of psychologists (the plurality of those responding) indicated that they use techniques from all schools of therapy.[79]

IPT assumes that current social functioning reflects past relationships and that resolving current issues will change interpersonal relationships in the future.

positive reinforcement — an event following a person's behavior that increases the frequency of that behavior

reinforcement — any event that increases the frequency of the preceding behavior

What is the Psychodynamic Approach for Treating Depression?

Modern psychodynamic approaches go by several different names, such as Ego Psychology, Object Relations, Psychoanalytic, Psychodynamic, and Neo-Freudian. All theories promote the concept that current psychological problems result from events in one's developmental history.

These schools of thought differ primarily in their theories regarding the role of interpersonal interactions in human personality development.

Psychodynamic Theorists

All psychodynamic theorists explain depression's origin based on personality development and its interaction with environmental events. In particular, Freud noted that depressed individuals seemed to experience an emotion similar to grief, except that they were more self-judgmental and their self-image tended to be negative. He suggested that contrary to grief (in which a person has experienced an actual traumatic loss of a loved one), the depressed person suffers because of a perceived internal loss to the self.

For example, children who are rejected or ignored by their mother might frequently feel anger or rage at this treatment. As adults, they lose their mother's physical presence, but she is still emotionally present as an internalized representation. In this case, the depressed person's self-criticism reflects an internalized anger toward the abandonment by the mother.

Clinicians often call this theory the "anger turned inward hypothesis" of depression.

Object Relations Theorists

More contemporary psychodynamic theorists, most notably those classified as *object relations* theorists, have developed these initial themes in different ways. These theorists refer to the self as the "subject" and other people as "objects." The subject internalizes "objects" and views them within the self as the image or representation of a significant other, most frequently the primary caregiver or "love object."

object relations—"objects" are the internal representation of "others," who are the focus of love or affection; the present or past relationships with these internalized love objects

Blatt, a prominent object relations theorist, also focuses on the theme of loss as part of the origin of depression.[81] Blatt distinguishes "*anaclitic depression*" from "*introjective depression*," describing how depression develops and manifests itself clinically, based on whether or not the patient's identity remains at the symbiosis level.

anaclitic depression—depressive feelings of abandonment based on the real or perceived loss of one's significant caretaker from childhood

introjective depression—anger toward one's parents that couldn't be expressed for fear of rejection and thus results in punitive reactions towards one's self

symbiotic — self and other are perceived as the same

Anaclitic Depression — This type of depression develops when impairment has occurred during the early stage of development, when the child was still in a *symbiotic* relationship with the caregiver and had not yet separated as a distinct identity. As an adult, the person is still stuck at this stage and will fear being abandoned and unloved. Feelings of separateness and anger cannot be expressed directly lest the loved object abandon the person. Consequently, this type of depression is theoretically characterized by feelings of helplessness, weakness, desire to be protected and cared for, and intense fear of loss/abandonment.

The presence of guilt and shame distinguishes anaclitic from introjective depression. Persons at the symbiotic development stage have no conceptualization of others and thus no internalized social expectations. They perceive everything as happening to themselves.

Guilt is not part of the pattern for anaclitic depression, because guilt is a result of a later developmental stage in which there are internalized social expectations.

Introjective Depression — This form of illness occurs in people who are thought to be past the stage of symbiosis, but have suffered impairment in their ability to separate and individuate from the primary caregiver (love object). As children, when they began to separate and act individually from their love object, they learned that this was not considered good or acceptable by the love object. Thus, as adults, they tend to feel they are unlovable and view resolution of the separation/individuation stage as tantamount to disloyalty; it is "bad" and unworthy of the high ideals that the *superego* imposes on them. The superego in persons with this kind of depression is well developed and is typically harsh, controlling, and committed to high and often unrealistic ideals. They expect themselves to perform at 100 percent without consideration for normal patterns of struggle and conflict in relationships.

superego — conscience, internalized societal norms

Individuals with this type of depression experience intense feelings of guilt, inferiority, and a constant sense of failure. They often spend much of their time trying to make up for their failings and are excessively concerned with receiving approval and recognition from the love object since this helps them feel "good" or "worthy."

Those with introjective depression might be very self-critical if they fail to meet others' expectations, or if they hurt someone else's feelings.

Psychodynamic Treatment Methods

Although object relations, ego psychology, and neo-Freudian approaches may differ in theory regarding the origin of depression, they are similar in treatment implementation.

In traditional psychodynamic therapy, the clinician attempts to present a "blank screen" to the patient, representing an attempt to appear neutral and objective yet giving no outside direction to the patient's thinking. The patient projects pressing issues and themes onto a "blank clinician." As the patient talks, the clinician listens for current events that reflect the historical conflicts and themes related to the current depressive symptoms.

The clinician responds by *interpreting* the patient's remarks to help the patient achieve insight or understand how developmental patterns shape current responses. The clinician's comments are typically open-ended and vague, allowing the patient to further respond without overt direction. The clinician's comments are also directed towards *catharsis*. As patients become aware of these issues, they can integrate this awareness into their ongoing lives and develop into emotionally mature adults.

interpreting — reflecting to the patient a clinical hypothesis regarding the connection between unconscious material and current or conscious material

catharsis — allowing the patient to experience, in the safety of the clinician's office, the emotion that could not be expressed as a child

If a mother was experienced as rejecting or cruel, the clinician creates and nurtures a therapeutic relationship that is safe and allows patients to express themselves without judgment or criticism.

At a later time, the clinician could point out the pattern the patient has been describing — feeling abandoned and rejected early in life, and then acting in ways now to confirm that rejection, while fearing to overtly express anger at being treated that way.

Throughout the therapeutic sessions, the clinician provides a relationship where the patient can openly begin to talk about feeling rejected and being angry without risking another rejection. Using the healing aspect of the therapeutic relationship, the clinician can counter dysfunctional developmental patterns.

For example, a psychodynamic clinician might sit quietly observing the patient who has just come into a session. This patient may say, "I just wanted to die after going to the grocery store because no one paid any attention to me. I'm worthless; I'm probably better off dead." As the clinician continues to observe in silence, the patient could become angry or even more despondent and say to the clinician, "See, you're doing it, too. I don't even matter enough for you to talk to me." At this point, the clinician could say something like, "Tell me more about feeling rejected." This allows the patient to get in touch with these feelings and produce other examples of perceived rejection, all the way back to the primary relationship with the caregiver.

Clinicians can use the therapeutic relationship to model interpersonal skills for treatment.[82–84] Specifically:

- **Modeling Negotiation Skills**—The clinician expresses views as tentative, open to correction by the patient, inviting elaboration and feedback by the patient to the clinician. ("It seems like this episode today might be related to how afraid you were to be angry at your mother. What do you think?")
- **Using the "Language Of Mutuality"**—This involves both the clinician and patient in a collaboration. ("Can we find other instances when you have felt like telling someone how hurt you were?")
- **Making Statements Rather Than Asking Questions**—This entails offering hypotheses about the patient's experiences and how they relate to one another. ("Your feelings of being isolated seem to affect your ability to work with others.")

Effectiveness of the Psychodynamic Approach in Treating Depression

meta-analysis — review of several studies with an assessment of overall treatment effects

The psychodynamic therapy was rated as the least effective of those used on most outcome measures.[86] Subsequent research has replicated these findings.[87, 88]

Literature cited by noted psychologist Hans Eysenck in a 1991 *meta-analysis* indicated that short-term psychodynamic psychotherapy was no more effective than no treatment at all.[85] This is not a new conclusion. A typical example of this research was a 1979 study involving 178 depressed individuals who were treated with 10 weeks of either insight-oriented psychodynamic psychotherapy, behavioral therapy emphasizing social skills training, amitriptyline, or relaxation therapy as the control condition.[86] The highest dropout rates in the study were for the psychodynamic and drug therapy conditions. Additionally, researchers found that 30 percent of the patients in the psychodynamic therapy group remained classified as moderately to severely depressed at the end of treatment compared with 19 percent in the control condition.

Research does indicate that modern psychodynamic therapy that is brief, focused, and uses more directive techniques than traditional psychoanalysis appears to be more effective in treating depression than a placebo or no treatment at all.

In one study comparing treatment methods, researchers randomly assigned 117 patients to either an eight- or 16-week treatment protocol with either cognitive-behavioral (CB) or psychodynamic-interpersonal (PI) therapy. Overall results indicated significant improvement in all patients, a result that extended to a three-month follow-up. Interestingly, researchers found no advantage to a 16-session treatment protocol versus an eight-week protocol. Their results indicated a slight advantage to CB over PI therapy. They concluded that the therapies were equivalent overall, with perhaps a marginal advantage to CB therapy.[82]

A more recent study's results indicated similar effectiveness for **very** brief and focused forms of CB and psychodynamic therapies. However, CB patients better maintained their improvement after one year.[91] Another recent study found that, after 10 weeks of outpatient treatment, a combined treatment group (who received both an older antidepressant and psychodynamic therapy) showed a marked reduction in depressive symptoms when compared with a group that received only the medication.[92]

Similarly, in a recent meta-analysis, psychodynamic therapy compared well in a direct comparison with CBT. However, the authors stress that the results may apply only to this specific, short-term form of dynamic therapy and do NOT indicate a general conclusion about the effectiveness of traditional psychodynamic therapy for depression.[93]

Although there is a clear absence of scientific data supporting psychodynamic therapy, this does not necessarily invalidate this treatment.[89,90] This lack of data may exist partly because such treatments are difficult to standardize and often have deeper therapeutic goals than symptom relief. For example, traditional dynamic therapy focuses on personality change (an outcome difficult to measure or obtain in a 10- to 20-week outcome study).

From The Patient's Perspective

I have been continuing therapy with Owen. Seems like I'm improving. I feel better. I had never realized how much guilt and unresolved feelings I've carried around about my mother. Maybe there are some good things that have come from her death, because I've resolved a lot and can get on with my life, instead of continuing to feel so worthless and trying so hard to please her. Work is much better; I may even get promoted. Ironic, since for awhile, I was sure I was going to lose my job. Terry and I are getting along better, but maybe we need to go to marital therapy like Owen suggested; we still fall into old patterns that make me feel bad. Got to go for now, Terry and I are playing doubles in tennis tonight.

What is the Interpersonal Therapy (IPT) Approach for Treating Depression?

Interpersonal therapy (IPT) recently gained attention after being included in the National Institute of Mental Health (NIMH) collaborative research program for depression treatment methods.[94] The assumption behind IPT is that the patient's current social functioning reflects past relationships. Thus, if the patient can resolve current relationship issues, then depressive symptoms ease and changes in interpersonal behavior continue into the future. Researchers initially chose IPT as a placebo, but soon found it as effective as *tricyclic medications* and cognitive therapy, providing significant relief for up to 70 percent of depressed patients.

tricyclic medications — a class of antidepressant medications affecting all three neurotransmitters described in chapter five

In a recent review, IPT was described as being derived from previous interpersonal and psychobiological theories with an emphasis on the interaction between biological and psychosocial factors in depression.[95] The authors noted that IPT does not endorse a specific model for the cause of depression; however, it does suggest that the patient's interpersonal relationships may be related to the onset of depression and may fuel a depression once it has begun.

IPT's focus differs from psychodynamic methods in three ways:

1. *Clinicians function as active advocates for patients rather than being neutral during sessions.*
2. *Treatment sessions focus on the "here and now" instead of past events.*
3. *Behavior between patient and clinician is explicitly not interpreted as transference (displacing of emotions or attitudes from the patient onto the clinician).*

In IPT, problematic behaviors are determined by early family experiences and participation in early social groups, both of which shape patient understanding of social behavior (e.g., "the world is a cruel place, so trust no one."). IPT theorists assume that personality plays a role in the development of depression through the way people handle anger, guilt, and overall feelings of self-worth. While theorists see these personality features as part of the predisposing factors in depression, clinical treatment with IPT focuses specifically on understanding symptom development and resolving interpersonal functioning. Clinicians deliberately avoid issues related to personality and psychopathology.

IPT assumes that clinical depression occurs in an interpersonal context and that the quality of the patient's interpersonal relationships affect disorder onset, response to treatment, and therapy outcome.

IPT theories emphasize that depression originates with the loss of social attachments; treatment focuses on that loss by:

- Resolving grief issues (e.g., loss of spouse)
- Exploring role transitions (e.g., going from being single to married, from homemaker to employee)
- Addressing maladaptive social behaviors by focusing on social deficits (e.g., lack of eye contact, poor assertiveness skills)
- Resolving previous interpersonal conflict (e.g., defensiveness, inability to communicate clearly)

IPT Treatment Methods

The usual IPT treatment course is 12 to 16 sessions with the stated goal of reducing depression symptoms while improving patient interpersonal functioning.[96, 97] Treatment involves three phases: initial, intermediate, and termination.

Assessment focuses on major areas of interpersonal functioning including grief and loss, role transitions, interpersonal conflict, and social skills deficits.

1. **Initial Phase** — Usually lasting from one to two sessions, the clinician educates the patient about the symptoms and effects of depression, and evaluates the patient to determine if medications might be helpful in treatment. The clinician then assesses the patient's interpersonal world by reviewing past or current relationships that may be related to depressive symptom onset and by discussing changes the patient desires in relationships. Finally, the clinician teaches the patient the IPT model and discusses practical matters, such as fees and scheduling appointments.

Clinician and patient develop an explicit therapy contract with set treatment goals.

Goals in the intermediate phase include helping the patient understand the relationship between depressive symptoms and interpersonal problems, exploring past and current interpersonal patterns, and encouraging problem solving to resolve old issues.

2. **Intermediate Phase** — Work begins on the highest priority interpersonal problem area. For example, a patient who is recently widowed or divorced may work on either grief, loss, or interpersonal conflict. The experience of losing a loved one may cause role confusion or a loss of part of one's identity. In addition, grief is often related to sadness, anger at the one who died, anxiety about the future, difficulty with concentration, and lack of energy.

   The intermediate phase also explores the patient's current and past interpersonal relationships to highlight maladaptive patterns. For example, exploring patterns of dependency might reveal how much the patient relied on an ex-spouse for instructions and help in social situations. The patient could then problem-solve ways to enjoy new independence and gain effective communication skills.

   Lastly, treatment in this area seeks to develop new opportunities to grow and form healthy relationships with others (e.g., recently widowed patients who do volunteer work or spend more time with siblings). This phase of IPT treatment typically takes the bulk of the time, lasting from six to eight sessions.

3. **Termination Phase** — Preparing the patient to complete therapy, this phase includes desensitizing the patient regarding periods of probable relapse and verifying the option of returning for therapy as needed. In addition, sessions examine plans for continuing to use what was learned in therapy to develop healthy relationships. This phase usually lasts for one to two sessions and completes the course of interpersonal therapy.

The clinician reviews treatment goals and progress made toward those goals, determines the patient's current assessment of interpersonal relationships, and facilitates the process of saying good-bye to one another.

In their book, Klerman and Weissman discuss newer applications of IPT to other forms of psychopathology, to groups, and in the treatment of other forms of depression.[96]

Effectiveness of IPT in Treating Depression

IPT has fared very well in studies assessing the utility of psychotherapy in treating depression. The NIMH multi-site collaborative study demonstrated that IPT was at least as effective as antidepressant medications and performed comparably with cognitive therapy. That study demonstrated significant relief for up to 70 percent of patients studied.[94]

Additional studies have supported the efficacy of IPT in randomized, controlled trials.[94, 98, 99] These studies demonstrated that IPT was superior to antidepressant medication in the treatment of mood, apathy, suicidal ideation, work, and interest measures, while drugs outperformed IPT on vegetative measures (e.g., sleep, appetite, and concentration). At a one-year follow-up, there were no significant differences between psychotherapy and drug treatment across all outcome measures except social functioning. IPT patients continued to demonstrate improvement in social functioning above that found for medicated patients.

In a recent summary of clinical guidelines for treatment, IPT is referred to as one of the approaches with the "... best documented efficiency in the literature for the specific treatment of major depressive disorder."[89 (pp. 4–5)] These reviewers also noted that IPT may be less effective than cognitive therapy for patients with personality disorders and more effective than cognitive therapy for patients with obsessive personality traits or who are single and living alone. Other authors reviewing IPT as a treatment for depression concluded that "... the data regarding IPT as a treatment alone and with antidepressants ... are very favorable."[95 (p. 234)] They noted that IPT appears to be effective as both an acute and maintenance treatment.

What is the Behavioral Therapy Approach for Treating Depression?

Research has empirically demonstrated that mood varies according to rates of pleasant and aversive activities.

The foundation of behavioral therapy is the concept of reinforcement. Reinforcement increases the frequency of a behavior and is measurable. Since reinforcement increases the rate of behavior, the depressed person either lacks reinforcement for healthy, positive behaviors and/or receives reinforcement for depressive symptoms.

Some individuals might feel a substantial elevation in their mood when they are at a party, while others might feel a substantial elevation in their mood when they finish cleaning the garage.

Pleasant activities can serve as a reinforcer in elevating mood, but depressed persons often lack the social skills needed for pleasant activities, or at least lack the ability to manifest these skills while they are depressed.[100] Therefore, one main objective of behavioral therapy is to increase the rate of pleasant activities and interactions that elevate mood.

Often, people with depression continue to engage in activities for which few reinforcers are available. For example, a person might work very hard and ignore hobbies or fulfilling interpersonal relationships, but not receive recognition for the extra work. Depressed patients have few reinforcers because of the combination of their own behaviors, their inability to create reinforcing events, and the response of the environment (lack of positive events).

One cannot predetermine what will be reinforcing to a particular patient; the only way to tell is to find out whether or not the proposed reinforcer increases the target behavior. For example, praising someone on the job may increase how long that person may stay at work (positive reinforcement), while the same praise may not affect someone else's behavior (no positive reinforcement).

Unwittingly, the supportive responses of family and friends may reinforce depressive behavior, and the patient's depressive behavior may increase in response. At least initially, the expression of depression can be socially reinforced by family and others, who attempt to support and encourage depressed persons. Unfortunately, this support can reinforce depressive behaviors, thus increasing their frequency and resulting in an overall decrease in the rate of positive reinforcement from normal life events. For example, when people show initial symptoms of depression (e.g., sadness, some withdrawal), family and friends may rally around and provide support and encouragement. As the symptoms continue, depressed people begin to cut themselves off from pleasant events (e.g., hobbies, friends, or dining out), which were part of their previous normal routines. Family and friends soon tire of giving seemingly futile support, a response viewed as rejection by depression sufferers. Soon, depressed individuals not only lack positive support and encouragement from others, but have very few reinforcers left from their normal routines. This situation increases depression and illustrates the social nature of the disorder.

Behavioral Treatment Methods

Treatment considerations center on the concept that depressed persons can learn to improve their social skills and increase their participation in pleasant activities. As people begin to experience an increase in pleasant activities and as their ability to relate well to others results in increased social reinforcement for non-depressed behaviors, their depression improves. Therefore, behavioral treatment usually consists of:

- **Defining a List of Pleasant Events for the Patient and Asking Them to Increase the Number of Pleasant Events They Are Doing on a Daily Basis** — This usually entails having patients keep a daily record of their activities, along with pleasure ratings of the activities, from one to 10. Pleasant event lists can also be divided into different categories such as social activities and accomplishments, with patients indicating high-reward activities that are singled out for special consideration.

Behavioral treatments for depression include:

- *Listing pleasant events and deliberately increasing them on a daily basis*
- *Rating mood during events at the beginning and the end of the day*
- *Conducting training on social skills, assertiveness training, problem-solving skills, and relaxation*
- *Utilizing behavioral rehearsal and role playing*
- *Practicing "in vivo" exposure*

Training Goals:

- ***Social Skills** — From greeting someone new to more complex communication skills*
- ***Assertiveness** — Responding to one's own thoughts and feelings without discounting others*
- ***Problem Solving** — Defining objectives, setting priorities, analyzing consequences*
- ***Relaxation** — Using deep breathing, imagery, and relaxation tapes to counteract depression's anxiety-laden, cognitive, and physiological impacts*

- **Asking Patients to Track Their Mood by Keeping a Diary of How They Feel During Events as well as at the Beginning and the End of the Day** — This exercise helps the patient and the clinician understand the relationship between mood at the beginning of the day, during activities, and at the end of the day. The mood diary serves as the basis for intervening, with techniques that help increase skills, reinforcers, and consequently mood.
- **Conducting Training on Social Skills, Assertiveness, Problem-Solving, and Relaxation** — Training in these areas can help patients build relationships, feel more in control, make decisions, and calm themselves.
- **Utilizing Behavioral Rehearsal and Role Playing** — Having patients rehearse and role-play new behaviors during the therapy sessions is often a powerful treatment approach. These techniques allow patients to practice new behaviors and receive direct feedback from the clinician. The clinician and patient can then discuss and work on anticipated road blocks to the successful use of new behaviors.
- **Practicing "In Vivo" Exposure** — *In vivo exposure* is the same thing as actual "on location" exposure. The clinician accompanies the patient to an environment typical of a feared social situation. The techniques practiced during the therapy sessions can then be practiced in the actual environment. This allows the patient to perfect the new skills and troubleshoot problems in a safe situation.

in vivo exposure — with the clinician present, patients practice techniques learned in therapy in the environment that represents the their most-feared situation

Effectiveness of the Behavioral Therapy Approach in Treating Depression

Many studies have demonstrated that behavioral treatment of depression can be effective and often superior to other treatments, such as insight-oriented and psychodynamic therapies. In one study, almost 200 outpatients with depression were treated with 10 weeks of behavior therapy, emphasizing skills training in areas like communication, social interaction, assertiveness, and decision-making.[86] Other conditions included a relaxation training control condition, insight-oriented psychodynamic therapy, and antidepressant medication. On outcome measures of depressive symptoms and social adjustment, study results indicated that behavior therapy ranked superior to other conditions on nine of the 10 measures used. This superiority held up on a three-month follow-up, where behavior therapy was still superior on seven out of the 10 measures. The insight-oriented treatment group emerged as the worst. Further, unlike the control group, a higher percentage of patients were still classified as moderate-to-severely depressed in the psychodynamic group.[86]

Behavior therapy has proven generally comparable in efficacy to cognitive therapy and pharmacotherapy.[89]

Recent reviews of relevant research noted that:

- Behavior therapy appears to be effective with depressed patients of all ages, showing good efficacy, efficiency, and endurance.[101]
- Behavior therapy and cognitive behavior therapy are equally effective.[101]
- Lists of effective depression treatments often overlook behavior therapy.[95]
- Behavioral methods are often included in other forms of therapy (e.g., cognitive therapy).[95]
- Relatively few recent studies have been conducted (e.g., behavior therapy was excluded from the NIMH clinical trials already mentioned.).[95]

What is the Cognitive-Behavioral Therapy Approach for Treating Depression?

Cognitive theories about the origin of depression focus on thoughts and images that are both internal to depressed persons and affect their behaviors and patterns of social reinforcement.

The two most influential of the cognitive theorists are Albert Ellis (Rational Emotive Behavior Therapy) and Aaron Beck (Cognitive Therapy).

Rational Emotive Behavior Therapy (REBT)

Albert Ellis is the founder and preeminent practitioner of REBT. The core concept of REBT is that life events do not drive an emotional disorder. Instead, how a person regards those events can produce emotional and behavioral problems including depression.

Practitioners describe this theoretical base as the "ABC Theory of Psychopathology" because **Activating Events** (situational triggers) activate **Beliefs** (rational and irrational), which are the direct source of emotional and behavioral **Consequences** (e.g., depression, anger, suicide attempts).[102, 103]

ABC THEORY

Activating Events
(Situational Triggers)
+
Beliefs
(Rational and Irrational)
=
Consequences
(Depression, Anger, Suicide Attempts)

Ellis states that human beings have inborn, biologically driven tendencies to experience both rational and irrational beliefs. These beliefs are defined by the impact they have on the individual. Rational beliefs promote a sense of happiness and ability to cope with life, and irrational beliefs promote intense negative emotions that impede the person's ability to deal with life events.

A depressed person might believe something that cannot be attributed to verifiable or observable data and is rigid and absolute. For example, patients who believe they are unlovable may not allow for those times when parents or friends have behaved lovingly toward them. In addition, they may interpret events in an exaggerated or unrealistic way. For example, a patient might decide, "I am unlovable," after going to the store and being virtually ignored by the

Several other factors distinguish rational and irrational beliefs:[103]

- *Verifiability (related to observable data)*
- *Demandingness (irrational beliefs are rigid and absolute)*

continued

continued
- *Evaluative conclusions (irrational beliefs produce exaggerated and unrealistic conclusions)*
- *Behavioral consequences (irrational beliefs produce behaviors that impede ability to function)*

According to Beck and his colleagues, the symptoms of depression (ranging from the physiological to considerations of suicide) are consequences of holding negative thought patterns.[104]

cashier. Drawing such a conclusion might trigger emotional consequences (e.g., feeling worthless or suicidal) as well as behavioral consequences (e.g., attempting suicide or avoiding close friends). Figure 4.1, below, illustrates examples of rational and irrational beliefs, all based on the same "Activating Event."

Beck's Cognitive Behavior Therapy

Aaron Beck's cognitive theories of depression are more specifically formulated than those of Ellis. He and his colleagues define a cognitive model of depression that hinges on three major concepts: the cognitive triad, schemata, and errors in judgment or thinking.[104] These concepts are described with examples below:

The Cognitive Triad—According to Beck, depressed people hold a variety of negative beliefs about:

1. **Themselves** — These beliefs result in self-criticism, guilt, and feelings of worthlessness (e.g., "I should never have left home as a teenager; I've screwed up my entire life.").
2. **The World Around Them** — Patients expect negative outcomes to their experiences and present others with demands that, because they cannot be met, become barriers to happiness (e.g., "I'll never find a wife; no one will ever want to marry me.").
3. **The Future** — Patients see the future as a bleak place because of anticipated frustration, catastrophe, and pain (e.g., "I'm a failure, so why try; I'll only mess up.").

Figure 4.1
Activating Event: The patient asks someone for a date and gets turned down.

Types of Beliefs		Beliefs
Verifiability	Rational thoughts are observable.	He said, "No," to going on a date.
	Irrational thoughts are unobservable.	He hates me.
Demandingness	Rational thoughts are flexible and malleable.	Maybe I'm not his type.
	Irrational thoughts are rigid and absolute.	Nobody will ever like me.
Evaluative Conclusions	Rational thoughts produce situation-specific and realistic conclusions.	The timing wasn't good for him; maybe he's involved with someone else.
	Irrational thoughts produce exaggerated and unrealistic conclusions.	I'll never find anybody that will love me.
Behavioral Consequences	Rational thoughts increase skills and options for behavior.	Maybe next time I'll find out more about the person as a friend, then I'll know more about whether or not to ask them out.
	Irrational thoughts produce behavior that impedes ability to function.	That's it! Trying to make new relationships will never work. I guess I'll have to be alone the rest of my life.

Schemata — The concept of **schemata** links various treatment approaches and is central to understanding personality disorder and depression.[105] Schemata represent underlying cognitive structures built up and elaborated over time, unlike specific negative beliefs usually linked to specific circumstances. Thought patterns can be activated by specific circumstances or triggers and produce consistent response patterns over time.

Everyone uses schemata to select information out of the endless stimuli in our environment. However, depressed people use schemata to maintain their negative view of themselves and the world in the face of positive evidence to the contrary. Depressive schemata are self-reinforcing because depressed people only notice those events that confirm the negative views and patterns. The stronger schemata become, the less able people are to "switch" them off and activate more reasonable, realistic ways of seeing the world instead. For instance, depressed people with a negative schemata might respond to compliments or praise from others by saying to themselves, "If they really knew me, they'd know how close I came to screwing that project up."

Beck is careful to point out that he accepts the role of genetics, behavior, and the interpersonal environment in the origin of depression, but ascribes primacy, to the role of thoughts in the generation of depression.[104]

Schemata can affect not only patterns of thought in the immediate moment, but can actually distort perceptual information by affecting attention filters and memory.

Schemata actually distort others' positive remarks and reinforce depressed people's feelings of worthlessness and isolation (e.g., "No one really knows me.").

Errors in Judgment or Thinking — The third concept in Beck's model of depression involves errors in judgment or thinking that occur when negative patterns of thought or schemata are active. These include cognitive distortions and other mistakes in analyzing information, such as:

- ***Arbitrary Inference*** — "Barbara did not say 'Hi' to me this morning; she hates me."
- ***Selective Abstraction*** — "In talking about our marriage, Bill said he didn't like my cooking; he is so critical of me."
- ***Over-generalization*** — "I got a flat tire; my whole life is a disaster."
- ***Magnification/Minimization*** — "My life will be ruined if people don't like my speech."
- ***Personalization*** — "These layoffs at work are all my fault."
- ***Dichotomous (black/white) Thinking*** — "I am completely worthless."

These cognitive errors produce intense negative emotional states because they are so rigid, moralistic, and inflexible to changes in the environment.

arbitrary inference — jumping to conclusions

selective abstraction — only attending to one detail in a series of events or stimuli

over-generalization — drawing a general conclusion from a specific incident

magnification/minimization — magnifying negatives and minimizing positive explanations for events

personalization — assuming outside events are related to oneself without evidence

dichotomous (black/white) thinking — extremes of idealization/devaluation

CBT Treatment Methods

Cognitive-behavioral clinicians focus on identifying, objectively testing, and correcting distorted thought patterns and underlying schemata. Using the active elements in CBT associated with change, a typical treatment approach would include:[106]

The collaboration process immediately involves patients in making decisions and taking charge of their own lives.

1. **Therapy as Active Collaboration**—From the beginning of treatment, the clinician emphasizes active collaboration and involves the patient in setting the session agenda. Usually, the clinician explicitly asks the patient what issues are most pressing and perhaps sharing the clinician's view of what could be accomplished in the session. The patient and clinician then mutually select issues to focus on during the session.

This phase involves teaching the patient about depression and the direct role that thoughts can play in improving mood.

Typically, CBT clinicians elicit more rational thinking from patients through questions that promote other alternatives and a recognition that the target belief was exaggerated (e.g., "Were you ever happy before you met Marty?").

2. **Educate Patients About Depression and the Treatment Approach**—The clinician educates the patient about the relationship between events, thoughts, feelings, and behavior, stressing that events (in themselves) do not determine emotional reaction, it is the thoughts about the events that give them meaning. (See the ABC model described in the section on Rational Emotive Therapy on pages 45–46.) A patient whose relationship is ending might think, "I can never be happy without Marty." The clinician might then use the cognitive triad to point out how such beliefs affect views of oneself, the world, and the future as well as how they contribute to depression. The clinician could then ask the patient something like, "What would your life be like if you realized that you could be happy without Marty?" This begins the process of testing belief validity.

This process usually results in a recognition that the belief was absolute or unrealistic and creates the opportunity to make positive change (e.g., "I guess I am right most of the time, but I do make some mistakes.").

3. **Build Hypothesis-Testing Skills**—The clinician would then teach patients hypothesis-testing skills by first examining specific beliefs that cause emotional distress (e.g., "I can't do anything right."), then directly testing these beliefs (e.g., have the patient make lists of what they have done wrong and right over the past three weeks), and asking the patient to evaluate the data.
4. **Increase Awareness of Thought Distortions**—This technique helps the patient recognize thought distortions (e.g., over-generalization). Clinicians use open-ended questions that elicit distorted thoughts and help the patient effectively test and eliminate these patterns. In response to a statement like, "I have always been a total failure," the clinician might ask, "Did you fail across the board or were there some areas in which you may have actually done well?" or "Have there been times when some failures have been worse than others? If so, does that mean that the partial failures were also partial successes?"

5. **Attack Schemata**—The clinician should help patients search for contradictory information to the negative schemata content and make more situation-specific conclusions rather than global assumptions (e.g., "I did poorly on that task, but I do better on other tasks." vs. "I am a failure.").
6. **Assign Homework**—Give the patient homework to focus on therapeutic targets, such as documenting:
   - Activating events that trigger certain beliefs
   - Feelings that relate to particular beliefs
   - Alternates to irrational beliefs
   - Evidence that supports or contradicts beliefs
   - "Absolute thinking" or "overgeneralizations"
   - Both negative and positive life events
7. **Utilize Behavior Techniques as Necessary**—Add behavioral techniques as necessary and indicated (e.g., increase pleasant events, provide communications and social skills training, use in vivo exposure, and conduct relaxation training).

One way to attack schemata is to have patients define qualities (e.g., competence) important to them and rate themselves on those qualities on a continuum from total incompetence to complete excellence. Most patients begin to realize that their competence on different tasks fluctuates and that they are more competent than they originally thought.

One example of homework is assigning the patient to participate in a "shame attack," a term coined by Ellis. The exercise pushes the patient to confront fear and realize that it is groundless. For example, patients who feel that they have to give in to others might be instructed to deliberately refuse some requests by friends and then to notice that the friendships did not end.

Effectiveness of Cognitive-Behavior Therapy in Treating Depression

Both REBT and cognitive-behavior therapy (CBT) have proved highly effective in treating depression. In the original meta-analysis of therapeutic outcome, REBT ranked second in producing the largest improvement in patients among the 10 forms of psychotherapy studied.[107] Another review of 70 REBT outcome studies concluded that after REBT, patients improved significantly compared to those placed on a waiting list for the same time.[108]

Researchers have found CBT to be at least as effective (and sometimes more effective) than medication, especially when relapse and dropout rates are considered. Several meta-analytic studies and other research have concluded that CBT is significantly more effective in treating depression than no treatment and was more effective than other forms of psychotherapy.[94, 109, 110] A recent review concluded that:[96]

- Beck's CBT is the most extensively evaluated psychosocial treatment for depression.
- CBT may need to be combined with medication for optimum effectiveness with severely depressed patients.[111]
- To achieve maximal effectiveness, clinicians need to be well trained in CBT due to the treatment complexity.

Other authors noted that CBT has been equal to or more effective than medications, and its effect has generally been at least as large or larger than other forms of psychotherapy.[89]

Rational Emotive Therapy steps parallel typical CBT treatment method by:

1. Forcefully disputing problematic beliefs
2. Engaging the patient to search for observable evidence to validate beliefs
3. Getting the patient to consider alternative explanations for situations
4. Giving homework
5. Utilizing in vivo exposure

Many of the outcome studies in which CBT has been found to be effective are described in chapter five in a summary of comparison studies between psychotherapy and antidepressant medication.

CBT has also been effective in treating "mild" to "severe" depression.[112–114]

How Does Group Therapy Help Those Suffering from Depression?

In this era of managed health care and health care reform, using group psychotherapy to treat depression can be cost-effective as well as therapeutically useful. There are well-developed guidelines describing the logistics and screening documents used to manage groups.[116, 117]

Group therapy is a common form of treatment for depression. Yalom has defined a set of 11 therapeutic factors that probably operate in one form or another in all groups.[116] Some researchers point out that several factors appear especially relevant in the treatment of major depression. These are Universality, Instillation of Hope, Interpersonal Learning, and Altruism.[118] The following discussion will explain how these and other factors enhance treatment.

- **Universality** — The awareness that other patients suffer similar symptoms and the growing understanding that depression is widespread help to break down the patient's feelings of loneliness and isolation.
- **Altruism** — In a group, depressed patients come to realize that they have something to contribute to others. By helping others, they begin to regain a sense of self-worth. Altruism has an important place in CB groups, namely that as patients help to correct distorted beliefs held by their peers, they are simultaneously correcting and testing their own cognitive distortions.[112]
- **Instillation of Hope** — Because hopelessness is a central feature of depression and suicidal ideation, patients in a group witness their peers' progress and learn that depression is not endless. This creates a sense of hope, which assists recovery.
- **Interpersonal Learning** — The interpersonal learning that occurs in a group setting challenges the interpersonal struggles inherent in depression. Patients learn how they participate in pushing others away and learn ways to reconnect with peers in the group and (by extension) with important people in their lives outside the group.

Treatment methods discussed in this section focus on cognitive-behavioral group therapy and interpersonal/psychodynamic groups.

Yalom's Therapeutic Factors of Groups are:[115]

1. *Instillation Of Hope*
2. *Universality*
3. *Imparting Of Information*
4. *Altruism*
5. *The Corrective Recapitulation of The Family Group*
6. *Development of Socialization Techniques*
7. *Imitative Behavior*
8. *Interpersonal Learning*
9. *Group Cohesiveness*
10. *Catharsis*
11. *Existential Factors*

The adult course, "Coping with Depression," comes with well-developed manuals for both instructors and participants. The course takes patients through behavioral techniques to improve mood (pleasant events, relaxation) as well as cognitive therapy techniques. Homework assignments are provided and reviewed as part of the treatment.[117] *In psychodynamic groups, there are no homework assignments or exercises.*

Cognitive-Behavioral (CB) Group Therapy

Time-limited and homogeneous groups are the most common among CB therapy groups. In this format, all group members are similarly diagnosed. They begin and end the group simultaneously, and membership is fixed for the duration of the group.

These groups are typically time-limited with a specific number of sessions and are highly structured, with clinicians playing a directive and active role throughout the therapy.

Early group meetings tend to focus on behavioral techniques designed to increase mood by addressing problems of inertia, passivity, or apathy. This not only improves mood, but as patients begin to experience some successes through the behavioral homework, group leaders challenge thoughts about failure, incompetence, and inability to succeed.

As the group progresses, clinicians provide techniques for correcting cognitive distortions. Additionally, the presence of "objective" peers facilitates the testing of distorted beliefs. For example, some patients might believe they are complete failures in life. As group therapy progresses and this belief is uncovered, those patients' peers have the opportunity to argue and test this belief.

Feedback from the group that corrects cognitive distortions is of powerful therapeutic value.

Interactional or Psychodynamic Group Therapy

Interactional or psychodynamic groups differ primarily because they function better with patients holding a wide variety of diagnoses. While CB groups are structured and directed by active clinician-leaders, dynamic groups are more loosely structured and would be at risk for "disabling inertia, a failure of spontaneous social interaction, and the possible escalation of symptoms."[118]

Groups with diverse perspectives and defense styles will form their own social system as members interact, and patients will engage in the same interactional patterns that pose problems for them outside the group.

Group leaders make use of "here-and-now" interactions to point out interactional patterns to patients and provide opportunities to try new interactive strategies. For example, depressed patients may attach themselves to stronger, protective peers, and they may act in concert during the group. This pattern captures the essence of the depressed person's dependency and unwillingness to be assertive as well as the protective peer's tendency to dominate others. These patterns can be noticed and discussed in group, allowing insight and encouragement for alternate behaviors.

Effectiveness of Group Therapy for Treating Depression

There are few controlled outcome studies on group therapy for depression; however, those conducted have demonstrated that CB groups are superior to placebo or behavior-only therapy conditions.[112–114, 117–120] Recently published guidelines indicate tentative support for cognitive-behavioral and interpersonal group therapies; these guidelines include very limited data suggesting that supportive group therapy might also be useful.[89]

In the United Kingdom, a "swim, gym, and creche" group assists low-income mothers at high risk for postnatal depression. Preliminary results indicate benefits from exercise and social support group functions.

Use of Marital Therapy in Treating Depression

Studies comparing "normally" distressed spouses with no depression to depressed-distressed couples found that the latter's communication patterns were more erratic and negative. These results suggest that depression and marital distress combine to make the situation worse.[122]

Most marital therapy effectiveness studies were conducted in the cognitive-behavioral tradition, emphasizing communication training and monitoring feedback to each partner. One study comparing antidepressant medication to marital/family therapy showed patients improved earlier with antidepressants; however, the marital therapy produced long-term improvements in depression, participation in family role tasks, and increased satisfaction with the marriage.[122]

The concept that marital therapy is useful in treating depression may seem controversial; however, both the success of interpersonal treatment and the concept that interpersonal behaviors affect depression support this focus.[121] Some researchers report that the life event that occurred most often prior to the onset of depression was an increase in arguments with one's spouse.[123] Other authors have found that those with depression are more emotionally vulnerable to hostile comments by family members compared to people with other disorders.[121, 124] Research indicates a divorce rate nine times higher than that of the general population among those who have experienced a depressive episode.[125]

One study found that the lack of an intimate, confiding relationship with a spouse or boyfriend increases a woman's risk of becoming depressed.[126] Further research indicates that those women who reported having marital conflict demonstrated relatively little improvement after individual therapy.[122]

A review of marital and family therapy concluded that behavioral couples therapy (BCT) was equally effective as individual cognitive therapy in relieving depression symptoms, but superior to cognitive therapy in reducing marital distress.[127] They also report on integrative BCT, which extends the behavioral approach by emphasizing spousal acceptance rather than communication skills training. They conclude this new form of marital therapy showed promise, and more recent reviews concur with these overall findings.[89]

Key Concepts for Chapter Four:

1. Psychodynamic therapy focuses on how historical events and developmental aspects of personality influence depression.
2. Interpersonal therapy uses a short-term therapeutic approach that focuses on how current events, social roles, and relationships play a role in depression.
3. Behavioral therapy focuses on the relationship of reinforcement and people's behaviors, especially social skills, with the lack of reinforcement for healthy behaviors impacting depressive symptoms.
4. Cognitive-behavioral therapy targets the relationship between a person's internal thoughts, images, and belief systems and their behavior.
5. Most psychological treatment approaches seek to:[76, 128]
    - Create an environment of trust, acceptance, and respect
    - Use collaborative treatment interventions
    - Allow the patient a "safe place" to experience and then learn to manage emotions
    - Expose the patient to behaviors and situations they typically avoid
    - Initially focus on skill building and altering symptoms that impact daily functioning

Chapter Five:
Biological Treatments for Depression

This chapter answers the following:

- **What Genetic Influences Affect Depression?** —This section reviews research indicating a genetic component to depression.
- **How are Neurochemical Influences Related to Depression?** —This section reviews the role of neurotransmitters in the origin of depression.
- **How are Medications Used to Treat Depression?** —This section reviews the different classes of medications used to treat depression and their side effects as well as research on preventing relapse and medication effectiveness.
- **Is it Better to Treat Depression with Medications, Psychotherapy, or Both?** —This section reviews research supporting a combined approach to treating depression as well as the effectiveness of psychotherapy versus medication treatment.
- **What Other Treatments are Used in a Biological Approach?** —This section reviews the use of Electroconvulsive Therapy (ECT), exercise, phototherapy, and experimental treatments.

THIS chapter presents a review of the genetic and neurochemical (or biological) influences on depression and compares medication to psychosocial treatments. Other biological treatments are also addressed, including the use of Electroconvulsive Therapy (ECT), St. Johns Wort (an herb), exercise, phototherapy, and other experimental treatments.

What Genetic Influences Affect Depression?

Research indicates that genetics contributes to depression, primarily by predisposing some people's brains to overreact, neurochemically, to stress. Additionally, an individual's own personality factors likely interact with this predisposition, leading to depression. (See chapter one, pages 3 through 4).[129, 130] In particular, these genetic studies indicate that:

- Depression occurs more frequently in first-degree relatives of depressed individuals.
- If one identical twin is depressed, the likelihood that the other twin will also be depressed is significantly higher than for fraternal twins (who share only half their genes).

These results support that, the greater the genetic similarity between two people when one is depressed, the more likely both will be depressed. Using this information, clinicians can better evaluate someone's potential for depression and consider treatment options that have been effective for one family member as potentially effective for the patient.

Some authors argue that the actual proportion of variability in measures of depression tied to genetic influences is about 16 percent. They concluded that life experiences were the most statistically important influence on depression scores.[80] Clearly, both genetic and environmental influences are important in understanding the origin of depression.

How are Neurochemical Influences Related to Depression?

neurons — nerve cells consisting of cell bodies (or soma), axons, and dendrites

synapse — the space between individual nerve cells in the brain

receptors — membrane-bound protein molecules with a highly specific shape that facilitates complementary binding by neurotransmitters or drugs

neurotransmitters — chemical agents in the brain that affect behavior, mood, and feelings

reuptake — reabsorption of a neurotransmitter into the cell that released it

metabolite — the product of the metabolic breakdown of a drug in the liver or kidneys

norepinephrine — a type of catecholamine that affects central nervous system functioning

serotonin — a neurotransmitter from the indoleamine group, which affects central nervous system functioning and appears to moderate the effects of many other neurotransmitters

catecholamine — a group of neurotransmitters (e.g., epinephrine, norepinephrine, and dopamine) produced in various regions of the brain

indoleamine — one of a group of biogenic amines (e.g., serotonin)

Brain cells, called *neurons*, constantly transmit information to one another by releasing chemicals into the gap between neurons, called the *synapse*. The neuron that releases the chemical is the presynaptic neuron. Cells receiving the chemical message are the postsynaptic cells, which have proteins on the cell surface called *receptors*. Receptors have a specific shape that allows only one molecule of the corresponding neurotransmitter to fit, analogous to a key and a lock. When the chemical from the presynaptic cell enters the synapse, it can be picked up by a postsynaptic receptor.

Through a complex system, the postsynaptic cell collates incoming signals, perhaps firing off a message of its own or being inhibited to do so. Chemical messengers transmitted from presynaptic to postsynaptic cells are called *neurotransmitters*. Since the messengers between cells are chemical, they must either be physically removed from the synapse or destroyed before another message can be sent. The presynaptic cell reabsorbs much of the neurotransmitter that was released, thus clearing the synapse. This process is referred to as *reuptake*.

There are also enzymes present in the synapse that will destroy neurotransmitters that are not absorbed through reuptake. These enzymes produce waste products that are referred to as *metabolites*, which are often measured in research studies concerning neurotransmitters and mental illness. Although many neurotransmitters have been identified, the two most important in depression research are *norepinephrine* and *serotonin*.

The classic biochemical theory of depression is called the "*catecholamine/indoleamine*" theory because of the central role of neurotransmitters, such as norepinephrine (a catecholamine) and serotonin (an indoleamine).[131, 132] The theory stated that depression resulted from deficiencies of these transmitters in the brain, fueling the concept of a "chemical imbalance." To remedy this "imbalance," drug treatments have focused on increasing these neurotransmitters' presence in the synapse through either:

1) Blocking the reuptake channels, or
2) Inhibiting enzyme actions in the synapse (such as monoamine oxidase), which reduces the destruction of neurotransmitters.

Recent reviews note that, because of the complexity of the disorder, major depression cannot be explained simply in terms of a biological cause.[133, 134] For example:

- To date, no coherent theory has emerged that adequately explains how a biochemical disruption can cause the experience of depression.

- No matter which antidepressant is selected, symptoms improve over time for 60 to 70 percent of patients.
- Antidepressant medications currently used seem to work about the same even though they all have different, and sometimes opposing, mechanisms of action.
- Most SSRI agents are broad-spectrum medications also used to treat anxiety disorders, including obsessions and compulsions.

The catecholamine/indoleamine theory was first proposed after clinicians observed that reserpine, a medication used to treat hypertension, sometimes produced depression as a side effect. Further research indicated that reserpine acted to deplete levels of catecholamines in the brain. The monoamine oxidase inhibitor (MAOI), iproniazid (originally created to treat tuberculosis) was also noted to improve depression in these patients.

How Are Medications Used to Treat Depression?

This section covers the medications used for treating depression, treatment considerations, and relapse prevention.

Using Antidepressant Medications

The most common biological treatment for depression is antidepressant medication. Several major classes of these medications exist, including selective serotonin reuptake inhibitors (SSRIs), dopamine-norepinephrine reuptake inhibitors, serotonin-norepinephrine reuptake inhibitors (SNRIs), tricyclics and tetracyclics, serotonin modulators, norepinephrine-serotonin modulators, and monoamine oxidase inhibitors (MAOIs).

All antidepressant medications have the potential to trigger a manic or hypomanic episode in persons with underlying bipolar disorder. For example, one study found that as many as 40 percent of those with bipolar disorder had experienced a manic or hypomanic episode triggered by an antidepressant.[135]

This general approach to medication treatment categorizes antidepressant drugs as one of the following:

- **First-Line Agents** — The SSRI antidepressants have the lowest toxicity, least number of drying and sedating side effects (except for paroxetine, which can be moderately more sedating), and are fairly effective for most people.
- **Second-Line Agents** — These drugs (dopamine-norepinephrine and serotonin-norepinephrine reuptake inhibitors) might be used for patients with a personal or family history of positive response to these medications or when first-line agents have been unsuccessful. Of these, venlafaxine is most commonly used, but has moderate drying and sedating side effects.
- **Third-line Agents** — Tricyclics, tetracyclics, and serotonin and norepinephrine-serotonin modulators have more serious side effects as well as potentially lethal or severe interactions with other medications or foods. The older tricyclics may still be prescribed for chronic-pain patients (due to their analgesic properties) or when the patient has severe, treatment-resistant depression unresponsive to newer antidepressants. Unlike other agents, MAOIs have fewer drying/sedating side effects.

The drugs discussed in this chapter reflect the order that the evolving research consensus identifies as most effective and safest for most patients. In the drug tables included, the term, "Typical Dose," indicates therapeutic dose; starting doses may be lower. The dosage ranges given are for adults and may vary significantly in pediatric, adolescent, or geriatric populations.

Antidepressant Side Effects

Almost all medications have some types of side effects that are unplanned or undesired impacts of the drug on the human body. Antidepressants are no different.

Common anti-depressant side effects include drying and sedating effects. Drying impacts the mucous membranes of the mouth and eyes; sedating causes general drowsiness. **Allow at least four to six weeks before achieving a steady-state concentration when initiating treatment or modifying the dose.** In addition, the most serious side effects can result in toxic reactions that can lead to serious consequences (even death) depending upon the medication and the type of reaction. Toxicity symptoms include nausea, vomiting, tremor, irritability, and muscle spasms.

__Warning:__ To prevent drug interactions, professionals conducting intake evaluations should routinely check if the patient is taking:

- *Antibiotics*
- *Herbal remedies*
- *Certain juices (e.g., grapefruit)*
- *Any new medications since the last visit*
- *Over-the-counter medications*

First-Line Agents

SSRIs inhibit serotonin reuptake but only bind weakly to the receptor sites of other neurotransmitters. Side-effect rates vary by drug and interact uniquely with each person's biochemistry; no specific side effects can be reliably predicted for any given drug and any given patient. Side effects common to all SSRIs include sexual dysfunction, decreased appetite, nausea, fatigue, daytime sedation, nervousness, restlessness, and anxiety. Special concerns often involve:

- **Rapid Discontinuation (except for fluoxetine)** —This condition can occur when a person suddenly stops taking an SSRI. Symptoms persist for one to two weeks and include dizziness, headache, tingling, "electric-shock" sensations, and flu-like symptoms.

  A single dose of the medication can be used to rapidly block withdrawal symptoms before reinstituting a more gradual tapering off of the medication. Fluoxetine is not subject to causing these types of symptoms when discontinued.
- **Drug Interactions** — Use of SSRIs with other drugs may cause "serotonin syndrome" with nausea, diarrhea, chills, palpitations, agitation, muscle twitching, and delirium. **SSRIs can be fatal if taken along with MAOIs.**

Table 5.1, on the opposite page, provides an "at-a-glance" summary of key information for each SSRI medication.

A recent comparison of the effect of SSRI medications on 23 different areas of functioning concluded that, although specific SSRI agents may have relatively greater or lesser side effects, they are roughly equivalent in terms of effectiveness. The study also found no clear way to tell which medication will work best for a given person.[136]

Second-Line Agents

Second-line agents for treating depression include an SNRI antidepressant and a dopamine-norepinephrine reuptake inhibitor. The former, venlafaxine, can be thought of as a tricyclic antidepressant without the negative side effects of the tricyclics.[137] In the second group, bupropion blocks the reuptake of dopamine and norepinephrine in the synapse. Bupropion has low rates of both drying and sedating side effects; venlafaxine is reported to have moderate levels of both side effects.

Duloxetine is a new antidepressant in the same class as venlafaxine that recently received FDA approval for depression. Preliminary studies demonstrate that this drug is better balanced in its effect on both neurotransmitter systems than any other drug on the market and has a favorable side-effect profile.[135]

Table 5.1 First-line Pharmacology Agents for Treating Depression

Drug (Alternate Names)	Typical Dose (mg/d)	Drug-Specific Side Effects
Escitalopram (Lexapro®)	10–20	Nausea, insomnia, diarrhea, fatigue and tiredness, sweating
Citalopram (Celexa®)	20–60	Similar to Lexapro
Fluoxetine (Prozac® or Sarafem®*)	20–60** (Prozac® Weekly–90)	Agitation, respiratory complaints, headache, dry mouth, tremors
Fluvoxamine (Luvox®)	50–300	Insomnia (especially if taken in the p.m.), agitation, confusion, headache, fine tremor, dizziness, diarrhea; used mostly with obsessive compulsive disorder rather than depression
Paroxetine (Paxil®)	10–60	Frequent urination, constipation, sweating, headache, fine tremor, dizziness, fatigue; paroxetine also has higher rates of sedating effects than other SSRIs
(New Extended Release)	(12.5–50)	(Less side effects, especially those related to the GI tract)
Sertraline*** (Zoloft®)	50–200	Nausea, diarrhea, dry mouth, insomnia, fine tremor, dizziness

* The patent for fluoxetine (Prozac®) has expired; therefore, generic forms may be available. Serafem is marketed for pre-mentrual dysphoric disorder (PMDD or PMS).

** Liquid Prozac has high levels of alcohol (12 percent) and should not be taken by persons on antabuse for treatment of alcohol dependence.

*** Requires tapering off rather than suddenly stopping the dose to avoid flu-like side effects.[138]

Venlafaxine is reported to be very effective in treating depression, particularly with patients who have failed to respond to other antidepressants, including the SSRIs. It also appears to be more effective than the SSRIs in the treatment of severe depression and may have a more rapid onset of action than other medications.[137]

Special concerns for these second-line agents often involve:

- **Contraindications** — Venlafaxine can produce elevations in blood pressure related to dose, and bupropion should be avoided in patients with anorexia or bulimia due to possible seizures.
- **Drug Interactions** — Although no studies exist for the use of venlafaxine with MAOIs, this combination could produce serious, perhaps fatal, reactions. Combining bupropion with MAOIs can cause a serotonergic syndrome with severe toxicity.

Table 5.2, on the next page, provides an "at-a-glance" summary of key information for the second-line agents.

Table 5.2 Second-line Pharmacology Agents for Treating Depression

Drug (Alternate Names)	Typical Dose (mg/d)	Drug-Specific Side Effects
Venlafaxine HCL (Effexor® or Effexor XR®)	75–375 (75–225 for Effexor XR)	Nausea, headache, sedation, dry mouth, dizziness, insomnia, weight loss, sweating, diarrhea, weakness, nervousness, sexual disturbance (especially in males)*
Bupropion Wellbutrin® XR or Wellbutrin® SR; Zyban®**	150–450 (XR) (300–450 SR)	Dry mouth, blurred vision, constipation, sweating, insomnia, headache, dizziness, hypertension, nausea/diarrhea

* The downside of venlafaxine is that it must be tapered off, not suddenly stopped, to avoid flu-like side effects.[138]

** Zyban is the name for bupropion when used for smoking cessation.

XR = Extended Release; SR = Sustained Release

Table 5.3, on pages 60–61, provides an "at-a-glance" summary of key information for these third-line agents.

Stopping these medications abruptly or large increases in dose can cause a syndrome with anxiety, fever, sweating, inflammation of the nasal mucosa, malaise, and other symptoms.

tardive dyskinesia — side effects of medications that cause annoying, mostly uncontrollable movements and include repetitive sucking or blinking, slow twisting of the hands, or other movements of the face and limbs

Third-Line Agents

Third-line agents for treating depression are the tricyclics and tetracyclics, serotonin modulators, norepinephrine-serotonin modulators, and monamine oxidase inhibitors (MAOIs).

Tricyclics/Tetracyclics — These drugs are broad-spectrum agents, which increase the availability of norepinephrine, serotonin, and dopamine in the synapse by reuptake blockade. In addition, they affect many different systems, which accounts for a high rate of side effects (including toxicity). While all the tricyclics/tetracyclics have a much higher rate of drying and sedating side effects than other classes of drugs, a few have a more moderate or low impact in these areas, specifically:

- **Clomipramine**: moderately sedating
- **Imipramine**: moderately drying and sedating
- **Nortriptyline**: moderately drying and sedating
- **Protriptyline**: low risk of sedating effects
- **Amoxapine**: moderately drying and sedating

Special concerns for all tricyclics/tetracyclics include:

- **Toxicity** — With all these drugs, the therapeutic dose is close to the toxic dose. Toxic symptoms are mostly anti-cholinergic (dry mouth, blurred vision, constipation, sweating, delayed urination). Next most common toxic symptoms are drowsiness, sedation, insomnia, excitement, disorientation/confusion, or headache. With tetracyclics, there is an added risk of dopamine antagonist side effects such as *tardive dyskinesia*.
- **Contraindications** — Avoid for suicidal patients and those at risk for seizures as these drugs may lower seizure threshold. Avoid using tetracyclics in patients at risk for alcohol/sedative withdrawal syndrome.

- **Drug Interactions** — There are many interactions with other medications, especially some SSRIs due to breakdown in the liver. Also, when prescribed with an SSRI, clinicians must monitor tricyclic levels carefully for potential *arrhythmia*.

arrhythmia — an irregularity in the normal rhythm or force of the heart beat

Serotonin Modulator (Trazadone) — This drug inhibits presynaptic serotonin reuptake and blocks postsynaptic serotonin receptors. While trazadone preserves normal sleep patterns and avoids the sexual side effects that often accompany SSRI use, it requires twice-daily dosing and titrating the dose.

Trazadone has low drying and moderate sedating effects and is typically prescribed at low doses (about 50 mg) as a sleep aid.

Norepinephrine-Serotonin Modulator (Mirtazapine) — This is a relatively new antidepressant that appears to act in a manner similar to venlafaxine.[65, 89, 137, 139] Mirtazapine requires only a single dose daily, does not cause sexual dysfunction, and has sedating properties, which attenuate over time (may be useful in treating depressed patients with marked insomnia). Drying is low to moderate in degree; the drug is sedating to a moderate degree.

Monoamine Oxidase Inhibitors (MAOIs) (Phenelzine, Tranylcypromine) — These drugs inhibit the enzyme, monamine oxidase, in the central nervous system, intestinal track, and platelets. MAOIs tend to be neither drying nor sedating.

There is a new, reversible MAOI, linezolid (Zyvox®), which is approved for use as an antibiotic/antimicrobial drug with all the same precautions about food and drug interactions as other MAOIs.

The MAOI, moclobemide, is available in Europe, but not in the United States. Moclobemide is more reversible; it doesn't inhibit neurotransmission for as long as other MAOIs.

Special concerns for MAOI use include:

- **Risk of Use with Foods Containing Tyramine or Over-the-Counter Medications** — Foods containing tyramine and non-prescription drugs (e.g., cold remedies, anti-asthma medications, and vitamin supplements) can cause a high-blood-pressure crisis indicated by headache, neck stiffness, nausea, vomiting, sweating (with fever or clammy skin), dilated pupils, photophobia, sudden nose bleed, chest pain, and either rapid or slow heartbeat.
- **Dosage Change** — Overdoses can be fatal; changing to another antidepressant requires 10 days without medication. Withdrawal symptoms are likely if MAOI is stopped abruptly.
- **Drug Interactions** — Combining MAOIs and SSRIs can be fatal.

Tyramine-rich foods include aged cheese, meat extracts, and sausage.

Selecting an Antidepressant Medication

Because of the high rate (30 to 50 percent) of patient nonresponse to the first drug taken, it may be necessary to try other drugs or classes.[140] However, for patients taking SSRIs, it can take up to a month to experience a positive effect. As a result, clinicians should avoid automatically changing medication too soon.[136]

Table 5.3 Third-line Pharmacology Agents for Treating Depression

Drug (Alternate Names)	Typical Dose (mg/d)	Drug-Specific Side Effects
TRICYCLICS AND TETRACYCLICS		
Amitriptyline (Elavil,® Endep®)	100–300	Dry mouth, sedation, weight gain, blurred vision, constipation, sweating, disorientation, fine tremor, dizziness, heart palpitations, noninjurious ECG changes, fatigue
Clomipramine Anafranil® (also Clonicalm,® used by veterinarians to manage canine separation anxiety disorder)	100–250	Dry mouth, blurred vision, constipation, insomnia, fine tremor, dizziness, heart palpitations, noninjurious ECG changes, weight gain, sexual disturbance
Doxepin Adapin,® Sinequan® (also Zonalon,® used by dermatologists to treat pruritis)	100–300	Dry mouth, sedation, blurred vision, constipation, dizziness, weight gain
Imipramine (Tofranil®)	100–300	Dry mouth, dizziness, blurred vision, constipation, sweating, delayed urination in elderly, sedation, insomnia, headache, fine tremor, heart palpitations, noninjurious changes in ECG, nausea/diarrhea, weight gain, sexual disturbance
Trimipramine (Surmontil®)	100–300	Sedation, dry mouth, constipation, confusion, fine tremor, dizziness, noninjurious ECG changes, weight gain
Desipramine (Norpramin®)	100–300	Dry mouth, heart palpitations
Nortriptyline (Pamelor,® Aventyl®)	50–200	Dry mouth, constipation, disorientation/confusion, fine tremor, fatigue
Protriptyline (Triptil,® Vivactil®)	15–60	Dry mouth, blurred vision, constipation, sweating, insomnia, dizziness, noninjurious ECG changes, fatigue
Amoxapine (Asendin®)	100–400	Dry mouth, constipation, delayed urination in elderly, sedation, insomnia, dizziness, heart palpitations, dermatitis/rash
SEROTONIN MODULATORS		
Trazodone (Desyrel®)	75–300	Sedation, dizziness, nausea/dry mouth, priapism (in males, sustained, painful erections lasting for several hours, possibly requiring surgery)
NOREPINEPHRINE-SEROTONIN MODULATOR		
Mirtazapine* (Remeron®)	15–45	Sedation that attenuates over time, dry mouth, weight gain, constipation, fatigue, dizziness, orthostatic hypotension; very rare occurrence of agranulocytosis; can increase serum cholesterol in some patients; **dramatic and serious weight gain that can result in health complications and serious problems with treatment compliance**

Table 5.3 (continued) Third-line Pharmacology Agents for Treating Depression

Drug (Alternate Names)	Typical Dose (mg/d)	Drug-Specific Side Effects
MAOIs		
Phenelzine (Nardil®)	15–90	Dry mouth, blurred vision, constipation, sedation, insomnia, fine tremor, dizziness, hear palpitations, nausea, weight gain, sexual disturbance
Tranylcypromine (Parnate®)	30–60	Dry mouth, sedation, insomnia, dizziness, heart palpitations

Other authors have noted that, while both the norepinephrine and serotonin systems have a degree of overlap (both are involved in modulating anxiety, irritability, pain, mood, emotion, and cognitive functioning), they are both independently involved in depression.[146] Studies indicate that patients may respond better to one system or the other. As a result, clinicians should evaluate an individual's unique responsiveness to different antidepressant drugs. For example, patients who have responded well to an SSRI may experience a relapse when serotonin, but **not** norepinephrine, is depleted and vice versa for patients who have responded positively to a norepinephrine reuptake inhibitor (NRI).

In addition to first-line SSRI medications, professionals may want to consider dual agents like the SNRIs. A series of studies suggests that selectively inhibiting both the serotonin and norepinephrine systems may target the broadest range of depressive symptoms. Thus, drugs like venlafaxine (Effexor®) may be more effective than a single-system SSRI like fluoxetine.

Several antidepressants now come in alternate forms (e.g., sustained-release versions, dissolvable tablets, liquid forms) that, while not representing improved effectiveness, may make administration or treatment compliance easier and reduce side effects for some individuals.

Most prescriptions for antidepressants and other psychoactive drugs (75 to 90 percent) are written by non-psychiatric physicians.[141] Given the current environment of U.S. managed care, physicians face rigid limitations on the time they can spend face to face with patients and ability to ensure medication compliance. A network of cooperating clinicians often offers better treatment coordination and followup.

Using a Treatment Algorithm for Administering Medications

According to a prospective trial published in the July 2004 issue of "Archives of General Psychiatry," depressed patients treated with an algorithm-based program had better outcomes than those treated with usual care.[142] An algorithm approach uses a sequence of treatment steps (either single medications or combinations) geared toward a more likely response or to achieve symptom remission.

In this trial for those with major depressive disorder, the Texas Medication Algorithm Project (TMAP) compared algorithm-guided treatment (ALGO) with treatment as usual (TAU) in four ALGO clinics, six TAU clinics, and four clinics offering TAU to patients with depression but ALGO to patients with schizophrenia or bipolar disorder.[143, 144]

Access TMAP's Web site for more information at www.mhmr.state.tx.us/centraloffice/medicaldirector/TMAPtoc.html.

Recommended Basis for Selecting Medication:

- *Prior history of suicide attempts, which limits ability to prescribe medications potentially lethal in overdose*
- *History of response to a particular drug or class of drugs*
- *Known family history of response to different drugs*
- *Cost*
- *Anticipated side effects and their safety/tolerability for a given patient*
- *Concurrent medical or substance abuse disorders, which could cause toxic drug interactions*
- *Other medications (or herbs) and potential drug interactions*
- *History of compliance with medications, indicating those most effective with the least side-effect intolerance*
- *Patient preference*
- *Scientific evidence on medication efficacy*

Although all patients improved during the one-year study ($P < .001$), those treated with the algorithm approach experienced significantly greater symptom reduction.

Limitations of the study included lack of randomization, lack of blinding of the outcome assessors, and varying degrees of algorithm adherence.

The TMAP has developed two algorithms, one for non-psychotic depression, and the other for psychotic depression. (See figures 5.4 and 5.5 on the following two pages.)

Preventing Relapse

Relapse typically occurs as a result of discontinuing medication use early in treatment as well as when symptoms subside. Recent reviewers note that 25 percent of patients who stop taking antidepressant medications following recovery will relapse within the next two months.[89] Possible explanations for the high relapse rates associated with medication treatment include patients failing to follow through and fill prescribed medications or stopping medications too soon.

Reducing relapse rates is a complex endeavor, involving patient education, duration of treatment, and consideration of cognitive behavior therapy following medication treatment. Educating patients on relapse risks and prevention strategies is vitally important as is the professional's awareness of the need to follow up with those suffering depression. Clinicians should recommend that antidepressants be continued for at least six months after depressive symptoms subside. Individuals having experienced two or more depressive episodes may benefit from continuing medications for years or even for the rest of their lives to prevent relapse.

Cognitive behavior therapy (CBT) may also be an effective continuation therapy following treatment with antidepressants.[89] Studies have shown that patients who responded well to CBT during the acute phase of depression and were then offered CBT therapy for the next two years had significantly lower relapse rates than those who discontinued therapy.[89, 145] These results clearly illustrate the importance of careful follow-up to prevent future depressive episodes.

From The Patient's Perspective

I am feeling better but not nearly as well as I want to feel. Progress seems so slow. Maybe I should try medications like Owen suggested. She says it will help me concentrate better and make faster progress in therapy. I'm afraid Terry will think I am weak if I take medication. Also, if I start taking medication maybe I won't ever be able to stop taking them. Owen says that is not true, so maybe I should try it.

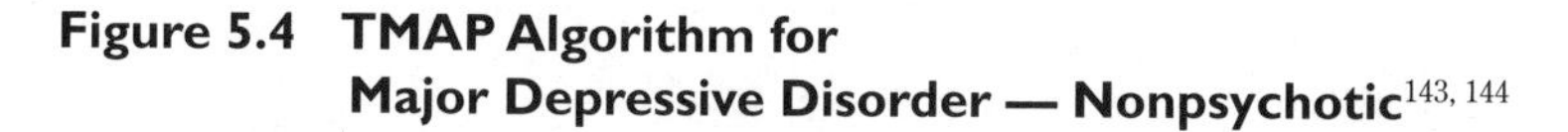

Figure 5.4 TMAP Algorithm for Major Depressive Disorder — Nonpsychotic[143, 144]

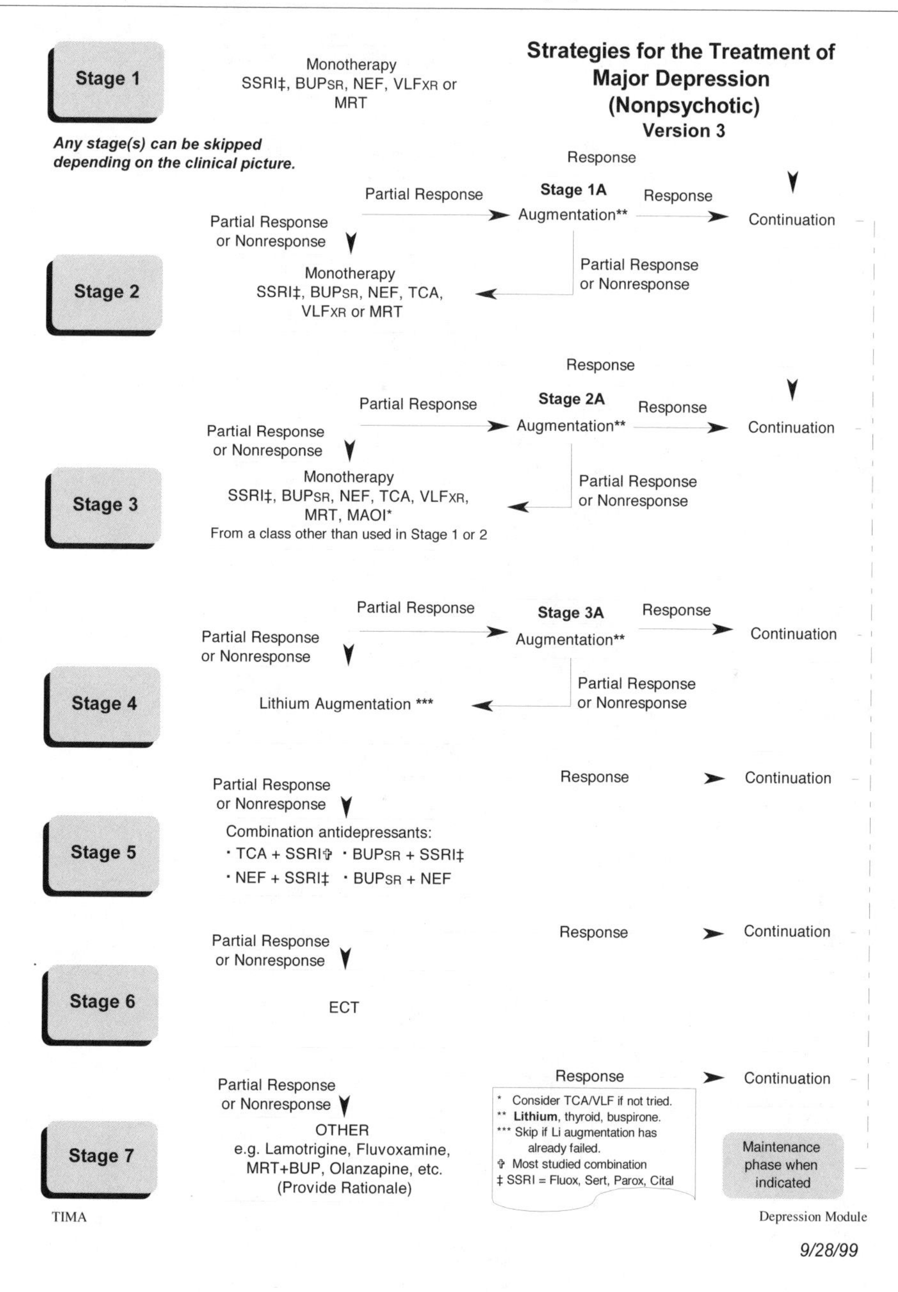

Legend:

SSRI — Selective Serotonin Release Inhibitor
BUPSR — Bupropion Sustained Release
NEF — Nefazdone (taken off market since Algorithm published)
VLFXR — Venlafaxine Extended Release

MRT — Mirtazapine
TCA — Tricyclics
ECT — Electroconvulsive Therapy
Li — Lithium

Figure 5.5 TMAP Algorithm for Major Depressive Disorder - Psychotic[143, 144]

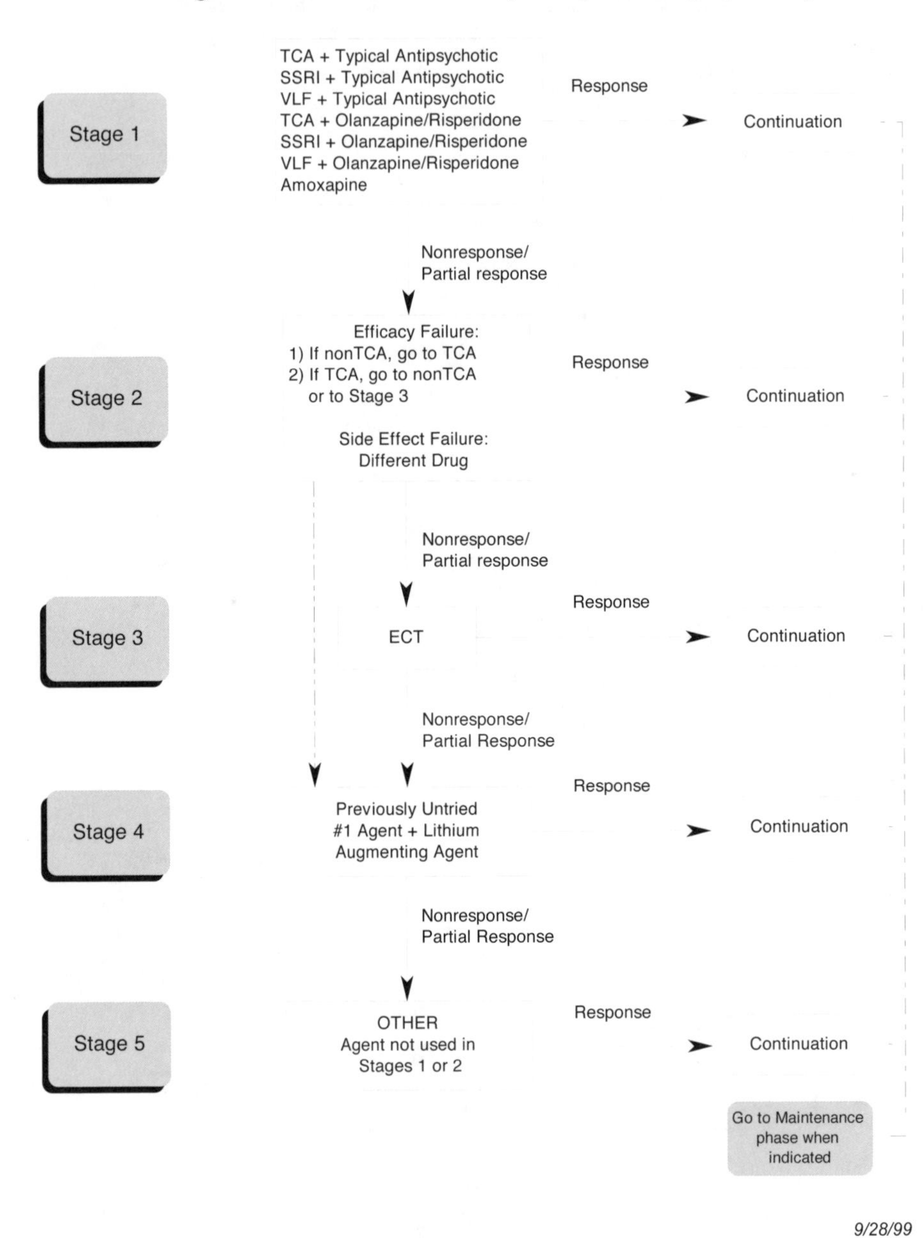

Legend:

SSRI — Selective Serotonin Release Inhibitor
VLF — Venlafaxine
TCA — Tricyclics
ECT — Electroconvulsive Therapy

Assessing Psychotropic Medication Efficacy

Substantial research supports psychotropic medication effectiveness for treating clinical depression by:[134, 146, 147]

- Providing effects that persist over time
- Demonstrating specific, positive impact on depressive symptoms
- Outperforming placebos
- Having effects that are not only superior, but distinct from placebos and from other psychoactive drugs such as benzodiazepines

Often a combination of medications proves effective, particularly a tricyclic and neuroleptic combination for *psychotic depression*. Researchers have found MAOIs effective for treating *atypical depression*, while tricyclic medications tend to relieve melancholic features, including weight loss, middle and late insomnia, and *psychomotor disturbance*.[131, 148]

psychotic depression — severe depression that includes delusions (false beliefs), or hallucinations (perceptual distortions, such as hearing voices or seeing things that are not there)

atypical depression — depression characterized by mood brightening, significant weight changes, mild paralysis

psychomotor disturbance — disturbance characterized by slowness in speaking or moving

Is it Better to Treat Depression with Medications, Psychotherapy, or Both?

Echoing the earlier discussion about whether or not depression results from a "chemical imbalance" or psychological processes, people often mistake their treatment option as a choice between either psychotherapy OR medications. However, substantial evidence exists that psychotherapy (particularly cognitive behavioral therapy and interpersonal therapy) and medications are equally effective in the short-term as well as promising for long-term success.[134, 149] Other important findings reveal that there is no difference between treatment effectiveness with regard to the severity of depression, challenging the frequent claim that psychotherapy, particularly cognitive therapy, does not work as well with severely depressed individuals.[95, 110, 116, 117]

Used alone, cognitive therapy appears to outperform medication in lowering relapse rates.

Patients who were treated exclusively with antidepressant medication:[95]

- Sought help more during the follow-up period
- Experienced higher rates of relapse
- Experienced fewer weeks of minimal or no symptoms compared to those who were treated exclusively with cognitive therapy

Unfortunately, the state of scientific knowledge about combined approaches is limited, despite this being one of the most common methods in clinical practice. This is due in part because of:[134]

- Complexities in carrying out studies of combined treatment
- Biases of medical and non-medical professionals

Recent Concerns about Antidepressant Safety

Many patients and clinicians alike became concerned when the FDA released a "public health advisory" in October, 2003 with a follow-up in March, 2004 concerning antidepressants and the risk for suicide in both pediatric and adult populations.[150] However, it is important to understand what the FDA actually concluded: that there needs to be stronger warnings about suicide risks, and patients should be monitored closely based on those risks.

- Overemphasis on highly controlled efficacy studies, usually either focusing on one treatment form or on a specific comparison between a medication and a form of psychotherapy.

The type of therapy practiced may determine whether or not combining medication and psychotherapy are superior to either used exclusively.

The research conducted to date includes a review of 17 controlled outcome studies, which found that combined treatment was only marginally better than psychotherapy or medication alone.[151] Another meta-analysis concluded that cognitive therapy was as effective as medication in the treatment of the acute depressive episode. This research found that combined treatment did not appear superior to either treatment conducted alone.[109] On the other hand, some researchers have compared interpersonal therapy (IPT) and medication, concluding that combining the two approaches is superior to medication or psychotherapy alone.[98] They found that IPT better relieved adjustment problems, such as: mood, apathy, suicidal ideation, and loss of pleasure, while medications better relieved sleep, appetite, and concentration problems.

Another advantage to the combined approach is that it covers all time periods of response (i.e., medications can produce a relatively quick treatment response, while therapy may help to reduce relapse rates once treatment ends). Disadvantages of the combined approach are no different than those of each therapy used alone.

Studies of combined treatment have indicated more effectiveness than using either psychotherapy or pharmacotherapy alone, but that the margin of difference between the two is small for mild-to-moderate depression; for more severe forms, combined treatment appears to be the best option.[152]

Clinicians may want to evaluate the degree of cognitive dysfunction when determining what form of treatment to recommend. One study evaluated the degree to which irrational beliefs and dysfunctional attitudes were present among inpatients. The results indicate great success treating those with high levels of these dysfunctional beliefs using a combined approach. Similarly, those with low-level cognitive dysfunction fared better with medications alone.[130] In addition, a large, multi-center study found that combining nefazadone and a form of cognitive-behavioral therapy reduced or eliminated depressive symptoms in an astonishing 85 percent of patients with chronic depression.[153] Just over 50 percent of those treated benefited from either form of treatment alone.

Additional research regarding combined treatment for depression suggests advantages and disadvantages for both medications and psychotherapy.[152] Figure 5.6, on the next page, compares these findings.

Based on this body of research, the best treatment in severe or chronic depression may be a combined treatment. In less severe, relatively uncomplicated cases, psychotherapy should probably be recommended (due to its decreased risk of side effects) followed by medication treatments. Whenever patients fail to respond to either medication or therapy alone, clinicians should consider combined treatment.[152]

Figure 5.6 Psychotherapy vs. Medication Advantages/Disadvantages[152]

	Psychotherapy	Medications
Advantages	• Lower relapse rates • Fewer side effects • Equally effective for acute depressive episode (cognitive therapy) • Found to be more effective for relieving mood problems, apathy, suicidal ideation, and loss of pleasure (IPT)	• Less time and energy required • Results occur generally in six to eight weeks • Effects persist over time • Good for those people whose personal preference is to "take a pill" to solve a problem • Cheaper in the short term
Disadvantages	• May take longer to see results • Takes more time and energy • Costs more initially; however, long-term antidepressant maintenance expenses potentially as costly • May be ineffective for those with a high genetic predisposition to the disorder	• Adverse side effects • Treatment dropout or non-compliance • Possible overdose • Discontinuation Syndrome (withdrawal-related, gastrointestinal or flu-like symptoms)

Some authors have attributed these results to the fact that combined treatment benefits all patients, whether or not they respond better to either therapy type; the combination compensates for the weakness of each approach used alone.[152]

What Other Treatments are Used in a Biological Approach?

This section covers Electroconvulsive Therapy (ECT), other biologically based treatments (e.g., St John's Wort — an herb, phototherapy —a type of bright light therapy), and exercise plus other emerging biological treatments.

Using Electroconvulsive Therapy (ECT) to Treat Depression

Electroconvulsive Therapy (ECT) induces a seizure through an external electrical source. ECT should be considered for those who:

- Have chronic or moderate-to-severe depression levels who have not responded to medications[89]
- Present with psychotic symptoms or catatonia
- Express preference for this treatment and/or have benefited from it in the past
- Express active and imminent suicidal ideation
- Refuse to eat

ECT might only cause death in .01 to .08 percent of those receiving treatment, while estimates of those diagnosed with depression who would have died (usually through suicide) without treatment are about 10 percent.[131]

ECT has a bad reputation as being a barbaric treatment for mental illness or depression, a reputation that is not fully deserved. About 75 percent of patients with severe depression improve following treatment.[8]

The exact mechanism by which ECT improves depression is unknown, but almost all neurotransmitters implicated in mental illness are affected by the procedure. The total number of treatments required for a full therapeutic effect ranges from six to 20. If there is no effect after 12 to 15 treatments, ECT probably cannot help alleviate the person's depression.[154]

ECT generally has been considered to be safer than many forms of combined antidepressant treatments. In general, risks do not exceed those associated with anesthesia. However, ECT may result in cardiovascular and neurological side effects; therefore, its use in patients with significant cardiovascular disease or increased intracranial pressure should be cautiously evaluated.[89]

Used correctly, ECT can be especially effective for those suffering from depression with intense suicidal or psychotic features.[155-158] One study noted that ECT was not nearly as effective for patients suffering from depression caused by stress or situational factors.[159]

Recent reviewers concluded that ECT has several positive indicators for treatment, including:[89]

- The highest response rate of ANY form of antidepressant treatment (80-90 percent of patients show improvement)
- Routine consideration for most moderate-to-severe depression cases where the patient was non-responsive to other treatments
- Improved symptoms in medication-resistant patients (typical 50 percent improvement rate)
- Potential treatment of choice for those suffering from psychotic depression, especially if unresponsive to medications
- Considered for those who suffer catatonic depression, have severe suicidality, refuse to eat, are pregnant, or desire a rapid antidepressant response

ECT disadvantages include side effects (cardiac arrest and memory loss) and higher relapse rates. Memory loss for what occurred during the days immediately preceding treatment can be part of an immediate period of confusion and disorientation that follows treatment. This usually clears up in a short time.

There is no evidence that ECT provides long-term benefits or that it prevents future relapse into depression. One study notes that about half of patients who receive ECT relapse within one year. If these patients are treated with follow-up antidepressant medications, the relapse rate drops to about 20 percent.[131]

Using Phototherapy to Treat Depression

Early trials in the 1980s suggested that bright light therapy might alleviate depression; however, these studies were challenged until recent controlled studies provided **preliminary** support for using phototherapy to reduce depression that has a seasonal component (particularly the winter "blues"). These authors also support phototherapy as a form of adjunctive therapy for those with chronic depression or dysthymia with seasonal exacerbations (Seasonal Affective Disorder).[89]

Reported improvement rates have been as high as 40 to 50 percent for persons suffering from winter depression after one week of treatment, but there is also evidence that relapse may occur if light therapy is withdrawn.[140]

Side-effects are fairly rare, but they can include headache, eye strain, irritability, insomnia, and occasionally hypomania. Treatment guidelines suggest that combined antidepressant and light therapy:[89]

- Increases the effectiveness of both treatment forms
- Should be considered in cases where neither therapy can be used at full dosages
- May result in photosensitization with some antidepressants

Using St. John's Wort to Treat Depression

St. John's Wort is an herb that has garnered wide attention for its purported antidepressant effects. **However, since it is not a regulated drug,** many of the preparations available to patients are non-standardized, making it difficult to know its preparation potency, to regulate the dosage, or to assure an impurity-free formulation.

Studies conducted prior to 2000 were generally positive about the effects of this herb; several review studies utilized double-blind, randomized placebo-controlled conditions.[160, 161]

One early study found that St. John's Wort was 1.5 times more likely to produce an antidepressant effect than placebo, and was equivalent in effectiveness to older tricyclic medications at least for mild-to-moderate depression.[162]

The 2004 Cochrane Review examined 27 trials of St. John's Wort involving almost 2,300 patients. They concluded that the herb reduced depression significantly better than placebo for the short-term treatment of mild-to-moderate depression, but that further research was needed comparing side effects over longer time periods and different dosage levels before it could be concluded that the herb worked as effectively as existing antidepressants.[163]

A review of prior meta-analyses of the herb resulted in a recommended dose of at least 900 mg/d to have an effect.[164]

Many authors also indicate that combined use of St. John's Wort with MAOIs is contraindicated, and the fact that the herb provides an antidepressant effect should argue for caution in any double use of St. John's Wort with a prescribed antidepressant. Patients considering this double use should discuss this approach with the prescribing professional.

Exercise is significantly more cost effective than other forms of depression treatment and provides myriad health benefits.

Using Exercise to Treat Depression

Scientists believe that exercise affects many sites within the nervous system and triggers the release of serotonin and dopamine — two chemicals in the brain linked to feeling calm, happy, and euphoric.

A recent review of exercise as a treatment intervention for various conditions noted that aerobic exercise can be more effective than a placebo and no-treatment conditions for mild-to-moderate depression.[165] These authors also note studies that compare the effectiveness of exercise to individual, group, and cognitive psychotherapy. Significant benefit can be achieved after approximately five weeks with supervised exercise sessions occurring at least three times per week. These sessions should consist of aerobic or nonaerobic activity of low-to-moderate intensity lasting from 20 to 60 minutes each. Researchers also noted that maintaining treatment gains depends on continuing activity for at least a year.

Using Experimental or Emerging Biological Treatments

A recent review highlighted several treatments that, despite being unapproved or in the experimental stage, show promise as an effective form of treatment.[166]

Originally thought to be the "pain neurotranmitter" that signalled damage to the body, Substance P is now viewed as one of the brain's central information pathways involved in experiencing pain, anxiety, and reactions to stressful environments.

Substance P — One of the best known of a newly identified group of neurotransmitters (neurokinins) is called Substance P. These neurokinins are found in the limbic, hypothalamic, and brainstem areas of the brain and are believed to function as pain neurotransmitters that mediate many other actions including bronchoconstriction, vasodilation, salivation, and smooth muscle contraction in the gut.

In animal studies, Substance P is part of the animal's defensive reactions to threat or trauma.[167]

Preliminary studies have found that agents that block the action of Substance P enhance transmission of serotonin in the brain. However, rather than blocking reuptake or increasing serotonin production, they appear to increase sensitivity of some of the brain's serotonin receptor sites.[168]

Studies in mice where Substance P has been blocked in the brain indicate that these mice were less anxious, more social, and less stressed by harsh environments than normal mice.[169]

Selegiline Patch — Administered via a skin patch, selegiline is an MAOI currently marked for use in Parkinson's disease. Taken orally, it often has the same significant side effects as other MAOIs related to gastrointestinal distress, but the patch seems to avoid these side effects. Early trials with human depression have been positive.

Vagal Nerve Stimulation — Another non-medication biological treatment is vagal nerve stimulation, which was approved in 1997 for treatment of refractory epilepsy. Preliminary studies of depression showed modest improvement (34 percent overall response rate in patients with treatment-resistant major depression) for a significant percentage of those who had failed more than seven antidepressant trials.

vagal nerve stimulation — a biological treatment involving implantation in the chest of a small pulse generator that sends electrical signals into the brain via the vagus nerve

Drug Development Based on the Stress-Response System — As previously discussed, the human stress-response is implicated in the origins of depression. Studies have shown that those successfully treated with antidepressants and ECT have reduced brain concentrations of *CRF (Corticotropin Releasing Factor)*. These studies link CRF and depression because preliminary results show reduced severity in both anxiety and depression.[166]

CRF — a peptide released during stress that sets off a chain reaction leading to the release of the stress hormone cortisol that can have negative long-term health effects

A potential treatment based on the stress-response system uses *mifepristone* to block hormones involved in the stress-response system. Preliminary results appear promising, especially for treating psychotic depression.[166]

mifepristone — a chemical that serves to block several stress hormones from affecting the brain

Transcranial Magnetic Stimulation (TMS) — This technique uses a coil placed against the scalp with an alternating current running through it, creating a powerful magnetic force that stimulates neurons in the brain. Although mixed results have been reported, a recent comprehensive review concludes that efficacy evidence for use with depression is "unconvincing."[170]

Use of brain imaging and related techniques — Recent studies have suggested that PET scans may be able to verify how effectively a given drug is producing an effect at the receptor sites themselves; this information may be invaluable in identifying which patients benefit from a given drug and dose.[133, 166] Similarly, a recent study using EEG technology was able to predict which patients would respond to antidepressant treatment.[171] As such technology develops, it will greatly aid the effectiveness of biological treatments.

Key Concepts for Chapter Five:

1. Although no coherent theory has emerged that adequately explains how a biochemical disruption can cause the experience of depression, researchers have identified two neurotransmitters — norepinephrine and serotonin — as the most important in studies of depression.
2. Clinicians administer antidepressants using basically an algorithmic approach with first-line agents being SSRIs, second-line agents being venlafaxine and bupropion, and third-line agents being tricyclics, tetracyclics, and serotonin and norepinephrine-serotonin modulators.
3. Side effects, often dangerous ones, can occur because the prescribing clinician has not been informed that a patient is also taking certain antibiotics, herbal remedies, juices, new medications since the last visit, and over-the-counter medications.
4. With first-line agents, side effects are typically less severe; however, rapid discontinuation (except for fluoxetine) can cause flu-like symptoms. Note: SSRIs can be fatal if taken with MAOIs.
5. Second-line agents may be effective for those unresponsive to first-line agents; however, these drugs should not be taken with MAOIs and bupropion should not be given to those with eating disorders due to possible seizures.
6. Third-line agents have typically had a higher rate of side effects; MAOIs especially can be difficult to take because of their potential fatal interaction with tyramine, SSRIs, and over-the counter medications.
7. Clinicians must evaluate side effects, contraindications, delay in experiencing a positive effect (especially with SSRIs), and previous response rates to determine the best medication strategy for each patient.
8. Combined biological and psychological treatment approaches offer a variety of advantages, including covering all time periods of response and preventing relapse.
9. Other biological treatments utilized with some success include ECT, phototherapy, exercise, and St. John's Wort. Experimental approaches currently build on what researchers are discovering about Substance P (a newly identified neurotransmitter), vagal nerve stimulation, medication administration via "patches," and new treatments based on the human stress response, physiological measures, and brain scanning technology.

Glossary

A

Aaron Beck — a psychiatrist prominently known for his cognitive behavioral theory and treatments for various mental disorders

acute suicidal risk — possible suicidal behavior within hours

anaclitic depression — depressive feelings of abandonment based on the real or perceived loss of one's significant caretaker from childhood

anhedonia — loss of pleasure in acts normally found pleasurable

arbitrary inference — jumping to conclusions

arrhythmia — an irregularity in the normal rhythm or force of the heart beat

atypical depression — depression characterized by mood brightening, significant weight changes, mild paralysis

C

catecholamine — a group of neurotransmitters (e.g., epinephrine, norepinephrine, and dopamine) produced in various regions of the brain

catharsis — allowing the patient to experience, in the safety of the clinician's office, the emotion that could not be expressed as a child

circadian rhythms — the daily regulation of sleep-wake cycles and activity patterns

comorbid — the simultaneous presence of two or more disorders

constricted — appearing apathetic and not displaying much emotion

countertransference — patient issues that trigger feelings in the clinician, such as anxiety, a sense of helplessness, feeling out of control, or feelings that may "echo" the patient's own feelings

CRF — a peptide released during stress that sets off a chain reaction leading to the release of the stress hormone cortisol that can have negative long-term health effects

D

dementia — loss of intellectual capacity in such areas as memory, judgment, and reasoning, usually due to brain deterioration

dichotomous (black/white) thinking — extremes of idealization/ devaluation

double depression — intense depressive episode that is superimposed on the milder, chronic depressive disorder called dysthymia

dysthymia — a persistent, low-level depression that has been ongoing for two years or more

E

equifinality — the theory that there may be many different pathways that lead to a similar clinical outcome (e.g., schizophrenia, depression, and autism)

H

hallucination — sensory perceptions without external stimulation; hearing voices or seeing things others do not; a compelling perceptual experience of seeing, hearing, or smelling something that is not actually present

hippocampus — an important part of the limbic system involved in working memory and other functions

hypomanic — exhibiting symptoms of mild mania

I

in vivo exposure — with the clinician present, patients practice techniques learned in therapy in the environment that represents the their most-feared situation

indoleamine — one of a group of biogenic amines (e.g., serotonin)

interpreting — reflecting to the patient a clinical hypothesis regarding the connection between unconscious material and current or conscious material

introjective depression — anger toward one's parents that couldn't be expressed for fear of rejection and thus results in punitive reactions towards one's self

L

labile — marked and rapid mood shifts (e.g., a client may smile briefly when asked about past hobbies, then burst suddenly into tears)

learned helplessness — passive behavior based on the expectation that one's efforts will fail

lethality — the probability of a fatal outcome, measured as the elapsed time between the use of the method and death plus the likelihood that medical intervention will not prevent death

M

magnification/minimization — magnifying negatives and minimizing positive explanations for events

meta-analysis — review of several studies with an assessment of overall treatment effects

metabolite — the product of the metabolic breakdown of a drug in the liver or kidneys

middle insomnia — waking in the middle of the night, often unable to gradually return to sleep

mifepristone — a chemical that serves to block several stress hormones from affecting the brain

mixed episode — a mixture of symptoms indicating both mania and depression

mood congruent — the content of the delusion or hallucination matches depressive symptoms

mood incongruent — the content of the delusion (or hallucination) does not match depressive symptoms

N

neurons — nerve cells consisting of cell bodies (or soma), axons, and dendrites

neurotransmitters — chemical agents in the brain that affect behavior, mood, and feelings.

norepinephrine — type of catecholamine that affects central nervous system functioning

O

object relations —"objects" are the internal representation of "others," who are the focus of love or affection; the present or past relationships with these internalized love objects

over-generalization — drawing a general conclusion from a specific incident

P

personalization — assuming outside events are related to oneself without evidence

positive reinforcement — an event following a person's behavior that increases the frequency of that behavior

psychomotor disturbance — disturbance characterized by slowness in speaking or moving

psychotic — impairment in awareness of reality, including symptoms of delusions and/or hallucinations

psychotic depression — severe depression that includes delusions (false beliefs) or hallucinations (perceptual distortions, such as hearing voices or seeing things that are not there)

psychotropic medications — medications that affect behavior, emotions. and/or cognitive processes

R

receptors — membrane-bound protein molecules with a highly specific shape that facilitates complementary binding by neurotransmitters or drugs

reinforcement — any event that increases the frequency of the preceding behavior

remission — absence of all symptoms; full remission if there have been no symptoms for at least six months, partial remission if no symptoms for less than six months

reuptake — reabsorption of a neurotransmitter into the cell that released it

rumination — thinking the same thoughts repeatedly

S

selective abstraction — only attending to one detail in a series of events or stimuli

serotonin — a neurotransmitter from the indoleamine group, which affects central nervous system functioning and appears to moderate the effects of many other neurotransmitters

superego — conscience; internalized societal norms

symbiotic — self and other are perceived as the same

synapse — the space between individual nerve cells in the brain

T

tardive dyskinesia — side effects of medications that cause annoying, mostly uncontrollable movements and include repetitive sucking or blinking, slow twisting of the hands, or other movements of the face and limbs

terminal insomnia — waking early and not being able to get back to sleep (e.g., at 4:00 or 5:00 a.m.)

tricyclic medications — a class of antidepressant medications affecting all three neurotransmitters

V

vagal nerve stimulation — a biological treatment involving implantation in the chest of a small pulse generator that sends electrical signals into the brain via the vagus nerve

Appendix:
Depression Assessment Instruments

THIS appendix provides more information on the depression and suicide assessment instruments mentioned in chapters two and three, including:

- Client-Rated, Self-Report Instruments
- Structured Interview and Clinician-Rated Systems
- Combined Instruments
- Suicide Assessment Scales

Client-Rated, Self-Report Instruments

Zung Scale and Center for Epidemiological Studies Depression Scale (CES-D)[172, 173] — These inventories are easy to administer, contain fewer than 30 items, and require 15–30 minutes for adults to complete. Each instrument produces a global score that is the sum of the weighted item ratings (related to symptom severity). Scores are interpreted on a range from normal to depressed.

The Zung scale covers five of the DSM diagnostic criteria for depression with four additional criteria. Some research suggests that the results of the Zung scale may be significantly closer to structured diagnostic interview results than the CES-D, which has mostly served as a tool for identifying depression research cases in community studies. Some authors suggest not using the CES-D as a clinical diagnostic instrument based on indications that it may produce false positive results.[37, 38]

Beck's Depression Inventory-II (BDI-2)[174] — The BDI assesses depressive symptoms based on DSM-IV criteria. The patient responds to 21 items covering specific thoughts and feelings experienced in the past week in the areas of cognitive, affective, somatic, and vegetative depression symptoms. Useful for those 13 years and older, the BDI can be administered individually or in groups, in a written or oral format. It takes approximately five to 10 minutes to complete and can be scored manually or by computer (a computer-based interpretation is available). The BDI is a screening tool for depression, with particular attention to items on hopelessness and suicidal ideation as the best indicators of potential suicidality.[39, 60]

Beck Cognition Checklist — This instrument assesses automatic thoughts related to anxiety and depression and has two subscales:

1. The CCL-A (measures anxiety symptoms)
2. The CCL-D (assesses depressive cognitions)

General Issues Related to Self-Report Measures

These instruments are typically "face valid"— meaning that it is obvious to the person being evaluated what the instrument measures. This is not serious in outpatient treatment settings, where clinicians also use other instruments to screen for depression, conduct follow-up interviews, and utilize other clinical evidence for diagnosis. However, in research settings, patients could exaggerate the degree of distress they report.

Coyne and others contend that most empirical depression studies using self-report instruments are, in fact, measuring self-reported general distress rather than clinical depression.[175, 176] Especially, in forensic settings, clinicians should always cross-check self-report data with other evidence.

A 1994 study evaluated the utility of the CCL with psychiatric outpatients and college students.[177] For the CCL-D, validity results were positive, and the subscale differentiated students from outpatients and outpatients by diagnostic groups. In another application of the instrument, medically ill patients were compared with psychiatric inpatients and controls.[178] The authors found that depressed psychiatric inpatients showed negative cognitive patterns when compared with depressed medically ill patients, who were best distinguished by symptoms of ***anhedonia***, low amounts of positive affect, and physiological hyperarousal.

anhedonia — loss of pleasure in acts normally found pleasurable

Geriatric Depression Scale (GDS)[59] — The GDS was developed to discriminate depressive symptoms from general characteristics of aging. Used as a self-report instrument or in an interview format, it has 30 items in a yes/no format that indicate depression. A short form of the GDS, developed from the items with the highest correlation to depression, has 15 items that require an average of five to seven minutes to complete.

A recent review of assessment instruments for the elderly concluded that the Geriatric Depression Scale (GDS) was the best-validated instrument for geriatric populations.[179] However, other reviewers noted that, in severely demented individuals, there was no well-validated scale; thus with this population, the GDS was considered unreliable. Instead, they recommended the Cornell Scale for Depression in Dementia (CSDD) for individuals with both dementia and possible depression.[180]

Structured Interview and Clinician-Rated Systems

Historically, the HRSD is the most common interview method for assessing depression.

Hamilton Rating Scale for Depression (HRSD)[181] — The HRSD was initially created to assess depression severity in those already diagnosed. It has become a common outcome measure for evaluating different treatment interventions, especially drug therapies and inpatient treatments.[182] The HRSD is a 21-item scale completed during a 30-minute interview. It is reliable and shows moderately good relationships to other measures of depression as well as being sensitive to changes in symptoms over time.

The HRSD has been modified to extend its usefulness based on continued use. For instance, both a computerized version and a paper-and-pencil, self-report version have been developed.[183, 184]

A recent study in a primary care setting related the HRSD with the Beck Depression Inventory, showing similar improvement rates over the course of treatment. However, the authors noted that, since the two scales emphasized different dimensions of depression, they would be more useful when used together.[182]

The Structured Clinical Interview for DSM-IV Axis I Disorders (SCID)[185] — The SCID is designed for use by trained interviewers to ensure a structured and consistent format for investigating psychiatric symptoms. Both the research version (SCID-RV) and the clinical version (SCID-CV) yield results based on DSM-IV diagnoses. They rate the severity of depressive symptoms based on the number of symptoms present and the interviewer's estimate of the degree of impairment.

The SCID-CV clinical version takes about 30–60 minutes to complete and examines only disorders that are frequently seen in clinical settings. The full research version (SCID-RV) takes 1.5 to two hours to complete and measures 32 different diagnoses, including major mental health and substance use disorders. The instrument demonstrates adequate reliability and validity for diagnostic purposes.

Schedule for Affective Disorders and Schizophrenia (SADS)[186] — The SADS uses a structured and consistent format for investigating psychiatric symptoms. SADS interviewers should be "highly trained individuals with extensive clinical knowledge."[38] The SADS is designed to evaluate current and lifetime affective disorders and yields diagnoses consistent with research criteria for studying depression, including other diagnostic categories. The instrument is a semi-structured interview divided into two parts and takes approximately 1.5 to 2 hours to administer. It covers symptoms of major psychiatric disorders, including depression. Part I obtains a detailed description of the clinical features of the current episode and during the week prior to the interview. Part II obtains historical information needed to confirm a lifetime diagnosis. It provides estimates of severity. The SADS was found to be more effective than the DIS in diagnosing depressive disorders.[56] However, the SADS has not been updated for DSM-IV diagnostic criteria.

SADS questions are progressive and have built-in criteria for whether or not to rule-out the symptom for current diagnostic purposes.

The Diagnostic Interview Schedule (DIS-IV) and the Computerized Diagnostic Interview (C-DIS)[187, 188] — The DIS is a structured diagnostic interview designed to be administered by experienced lay interviewers without clinical training. The computerized version (C-DIS) can be self-administered with an assistant to answer questions, if needed. The DIS has been used in psychiatric survey research for decades to assess the prevalence of psychiatric disorders in the general population. Modules cover mood, anxiety, schizophrenia, eating, somatization, psychoactive substance abuse, and antisocial personality disorders.

The DIS provides both current and lifetime diagnostic information.

The Composite International Diagnostic Interview (CIDI)[189, 190] — Similar to the DIS, the CIDI is a structured diagnostic interview for all DSM-IV diagnoses designed for survey research employing lay rather than clinician interviewers. It is most frequently used for research rather than for diagnosis when identifying depression cases for further study.

The SCID or the HRSD would better serve clinical diagnostic needs than the CIDI.

Cornell Scale for Depression in Dementia (CSDD)[180] — An interviewer-administered scale using combined information from both the patient and an outside informant (such as a family member). The Cornell Scale measures various factors, such as: depression, biological rhythm disruption, agitation/psychosis, and negative symptoms (e.g., anhedonia and poor concentration).

Combined Instruments

Recently, the PRIME-MD was converted to a patient-only questionnaire, which was found to be more efficient in terms of the physician's time and about as accurate as the PRIME-MD when used as a self-report instrument along with physician interviews.[192]

Primary Care Evaluation of Mental Disorders (PRIME-MD)[191] —This instrument recently received increased research attention and was developed primarily for use in primary care settings by physicians. The PRIME-MD consists of a questionnaire completed by the patient prior to seeing the physician. The physician then follows-up with additional questions in a clinical interview. Two questions on the PRIME-MD are specific to depression: one dealing with anhedonia (loss of pleasure) and another dealing with depressed mood. Responses to these two questions were found to accurately classify 96 percent of depressed patients in this setting.

Accurately identifying non-depressed patients can also be achieved with this instrument as well. If, for example, the patient endorses either of the screening items (anhedonia or depressed mood), then the physician asks additional questions about four core areas of functioning — sleep disturbance, appetite change, anhedonia, and low self-esteem. Patients reporting at least two of the above four symptoms correctly identified almost all depressed patients (97 percent) and also correctly identified non-depressed patients (94 percent).[72]

Harvard Department of Psychiatry/ National Depression Screening Day Scale (HANDS)[193] — In recent years, the National Depression Screening Day (NDSD) has been inaugurated across the country to encourage the public to:

- Become informed about depression
- Take a brief inventory to assess for depression (typically the Zung inventory)
- Have assessment information reviewed by a mental health professional and receive feedback

HANDS was designed for general applicability in clinical settings apart from NDSD.

Hoping to improve the efficiency of the screening day, investigators at Harvard created HANDS. All diagnoses using this tool were confirmed with the SCID. The final HANDS had only 10 items, but was reported to have performed as well as the 20-item Zung and the 21-item BDI-II.

Suicide Assessment Scales

Beck Hopelessness Scale (BHS)[60, 61] — The BHS measures negative attitudes about the future (pessimism), helps evaluate suicide potential, and effectively compliments other depression measures. The BHS is a 20-item, self-report instrument useful for adults age 17 and older. It takes approximately five to 10 minutes to complete with computer scoring and interpretation available. It outperforms the BDI in accounting for suicide risk. Scores of 9 or more predict eventual suicide (within five to 10 years) for those who are depressed and have suicidal ideation.

The ability of the BHS instrument to assess suicide risk highlights the link between hopelessness and depression.[60, 61]

Beck Scale for Suicidal Ideation[30, 60, 62] — This scale detects and measures the severity of suicidal ideation in adults and adolescents. It is a 21-item scale that can be administered to adults age 17 and older, individually or in groups, and takes approximately five to 10 minutes to complete with computer scoring and interpretation available. The Beck Scale for Suicidal Ideation has good validity and reliability and is best used for monitoring quality/quantity of changes in ongoing suicidal ideation.

This tool is especially useful in settings where clinical evaluation for suicide is unavailable or for clinicians not fully trained in recognizing suicidal tendencies.

Firestone Assessment of Self-destructive Thoughts[46] — This instrument was designed to assist in clinical assessment of suicide potential for adults age 16 and over. It is developed to be administered in a group setting and takes approximately 20 minutes to complete. It measures 11 levels of progressively self-destructive thoughts on a continuum that includes social isolation, eating disorders, substance abuse, self-mutilation, and suicide.

Suicide Probability Scale (SPS)[60, 63] — This self-report scale measure attitudes and behaviors relevant to suicide risk for people age 14 and older. This 36-item scale takes approximately five to 10 minutes to complete and can be administered individually or in groups. It yields scores on five scales covering hopelessness, suicide ideation, negative self-evaluations, hostility, and a total score.

The SPS is based on concepts related to suicide potential but does not assess known risk factors.

Scale for Suicidal Ideation (SSI)[64] — This scale has 19 items on which a trained clinician rates the severity of a patient's suicidal thoughts and plans. If the clinician detects any positive ideation of items four or five (active and passive wishes to die), all remaining items are rated. The Center for Cognitive Therapy considers scores of 10 or higher indicative of elevated suicidal risk that bears closer monitoring. Two subscales measure the intensity of patient suicidal ideation at the "worst" point in their lives (SSI-W) and "currently" (SSI-C). A 1999 study found that patients who scored in the higher risk for suicide ideation at the worst point in their lives had 14x greater odds for committing suicide than patients in the lower risk category.[194] However, the SSI-C was not found to be a useful predictor.

Bongar's review indicates that outpatients unresponsive to psychotherapy (who score high on the SSI-W and score consistently high on the BHS over time) should be considered at high risk for eventual suicide.[45]

Suicidal Intent Scale (SIS)[64] — This instrument is often used in conjunction with the SSI and measures suicidal preparations, planning, circumstances of a prior attempt, and the patient's reactions to the prior attempt (disappointment, etc.) to evaluate suicide attempt. It has proven useful to clinicians in judging the seriousness of a prior suicide attempt and estimating the potential seriousness of a new attempt.

Los Angeles Suicide Prevention Center Scale[66] — This scale was designed to serve as a clinical aid for evaluating patients (either calling on a crisis line or dropping in to a center), who have already identified themselves as suicidal. It is used in the Center to decide how to manage the patient.

Adult Suicide Ideation Questionnaire (ASIQ)[67] — This instrument consists of 25 items designed to measure specific suicidal thoughts and behaviors, rated by the patient on a seven-point scale that indicates how specific the thoughts have been. The ratings also indicate the frequency of occurrence of the thoughts within the past month. High scores are reported to indicate frequent suicidal thoughts.

Suicidal Behavior History Form (SBHF)[68] — This instrument was developed to assist clinicians in systematically obtaining information on a patient's history of suicidal behavior.

Risk-Rescue Rating Scale[69] — This instrument can be used to evaluate current or prior suicide attempts or plans as to both the degree of potential risk of the plan and the likelihood that the person could be rescued.

Lethality of Suicide Attempt Rating Scale (LSARS)[70] — This is an 11-point scale designed to measure the degree of lethality in a suicide attempt. It can be useful for evaluating how prior suicide attempts might suggest the likelihood of a future lethal attempt.

Reasons for Living Inventory[71] — This is a self-report measure with 48 items intended to describe patients' beliefs that may mediate suicidal behaviors. The measure has been found to discriminate between suicidal and nonsuicidal persons, but the scale's psychometric properties and cutoff scores are still being evaluated.[71]

Psychometric Assessments

In both inpatient and outpatient settings, clinicians regularly use psychometric instruments to facilitate diagnosis and describe patient personality characteristics.

Rorschach Inkblot Test -- The Rorschach consists of 10 cards with randomly created inkblots, some in monochrome and some in color. The cards are shown to patients one at a time, and their answers are recorded and later scored. This test is a "projective" measure of personality, revealing information that can be very useful in diagnosis and treatment planning.

There are many systems available for scoring and interpreting responses to the Rorschach test. The most widely used is the **Exner Method**, which defines a comprehensive system for administering, scoring, and interpreting Rorschach results.[195] Many consider this to be the best system to use for two reasons:

1. Its large normative base allows the clinician to determine how unusual a particular score is for a particular patient.
2. This system has survived a great deal of research on its validity and utility. Helpful indices are made up of combined test scores and help diagnose depression successfully.

Because the Rorschach is both a time- and labor-intensive tool, it is inefficient for diagnosis. However, this test produces information especially useful for developing treatment plans and understanding a patient's therapy progress.

Exner's Depression Index (DEPI) utilizes seven, key indicators drawn from the Rorschach's results. Exner indicates that individuals who score a "5" on the index share many features with those who are diagnosed as depressed, but the actual diagnosis may vary depending on history and presentation. Scores of "6" out of "7" indicate a serious affective problem.

***Note that** schizophrenics may often have a high DEPI score, usually indicating that the schizophrenic person is also depressed. A high score cannot be directly equated with a major depressive episode.*[195]

MMPI and MMPI-2[196, 197] — These instruments are widely used to assess individuals who present depressive symptoms. The original MMPI consists of 566 statements about the person taking the test (e.g., "I wake up fresh and refreshed most mornings," "It is safer to trust nobody."). Clients are asked to rate whether these items are true or false. The test is then scored, often electronically, and a profile constructed indicating test-taking attitude, clinical problems, and content analysis of specific scales. A revised form is now called the MMPI-2.

Both versions of the MMPI have a "scale 2" originally developed to assess symptoms and features of clinical depression, including denial of happiness and self-worth, physical and somatic complaints associated with depression, and lack of interest in the environment. According to Graham, this scale is a valuable indicator of the patient's discomfort and dissatisfaction with life. He suggests that very elevated scores (T scores above 80) indicate clinical depression, and patients with scores in this range often receive depressive diagnoses. More moderate scores (probably T scores in the 60s) tend to indicate a lifestyle characterized by poor morale and lack of involvement.[198] Moderate scores on this scale have also been found in individuals who recently underwent a major life change or transition, such as hospitalization or incarceration.

As with the Rorschach test, scores on the MMPI are not specific enough for diagnosis; clinicians must consider other information when evaluating the results.

Thematic Apperception Test (TAT) — The TAT, like the Rorschach, is a projective test that presents patients with a series of ambiguous, black-and-white pictures. Clients are asked to make up a story about the picture. The theory behind the TAT is that patients will project into their stories the prominent themes and conflicts in their own lives. However, there is no normative base to use when comparing patient responses. Despite this, many clinicians continue to use the test, scoring it according to the rules developed for the theoretical system with which they are familiar.

The TAT is not in itself an efficient tool for diagnosing depression. However, information gained from the TAT may help clinicians develop treatment plans and understand the complexity of the patient's life.

References

1. Gilbert, P. (1984). *Depression: From Psychology to Brain State.* Hillsdale, NJ: Lawrence Erlbaum Associates, Ltd.
2. Seligman, M.E. (1975). *Helplessness: On Depression, Development and Death.* San Francisco: Freeman.
3. World Health Organization. (2001). *Mental Health: New Understanding, New Hope.* Geneva: World Health Organization.
4. United States Surgeon General. (1999). *Mental Health: A Report of the Surgeon General.* Washington, DC: U.S. Government Printing Office. Available online at: http://www.surgeongeneral.gov/library/mental-health/
5. American Psychiatric Association. (2000). *Diagnostic and Statistical Manual of Mental Disorders - Text Revision (4th Ed.).* Washington, DC: American Psychiatric Association.
6. Regier, D.A., Farmer, M.E., Rae, D.S., Myers, J.K., et. al. (1993). One-month prevalence of mental disorders in the United States and sociodemographic characteristics: The epidemiologic catchment area study. *Acta Psychiatric Scandia,* 88: 35-47.
7. Nolen-Hoeksema, S. (1987). Sex differences in depression: Theory and evidence. *Psychological Bulletin,* 101, 259-282.
8. Seligman, M.E. (1993). *What You Can Change & What You Can't: The Complete Guide to Successful Self-improvement.* New York: Alfred A. Knopf.
9. Nolen-Hoeksema, S. (1990). *Sex Differences in Depression.* Stanford, CA: Stanford University Press.
10. Kaelber, C.T., Moul, D.E. & Farmer, M.E. (1995). Epidemiology of Depression. In E.E. Beckham & W.R. Leber (Eds). *Handbook of Depression (2nd Ed).* New York: Guilford Press.
11. Kuhl, J. (1981). Motivational and functional helplessness: The moderating effect of state- versus action-orientation. *Journal of Personality and Social Psychology, 40,* 155-170.
12. Levine, M.P. & Smolak, L. (1996). Media as a context for the development of disordered eating. In L. Smolak, M.P. Levine, & R. Striegel-Moore (Eds). *The Developmental Psychopathology of Eating Disorders: Implications for Research, Prevention, and Treatment.* Mahwah, NJ: Erlbaum.
13. Brownell, K.D. (1991). Dieting and the search for the perfect body: Where physiology and culture collide. *Behavior Therapy,* 22, 1-12.
14. Nolen-Hoeksema, S., Larson, J., & Grayson, C. (1999). Explaining the gender difference in depressive symptoms. *Journal of Personality and Social Psychology,* 77(5), 1061-1072.
15. Bierut, L.J., Heath, A.C., Bucholz, K.K., Dinwiddie, S.H., Madden, P.A., Satham, D.J., Dunne, M.P. & Martin, N.G. (1999). Major depressive disorder in a community-based twin samples: Are there different genetic and environmental contributions for men and women? *Archives of General Psychiatry,* 56(6), 557-563.
16. Robins, L., Helzer, J., Weissman, M., Orvaschel, H., Gruenberg, E., Burke, J., & Regier, J. (1984). Lifetime prevalence of specific psychiatric disorders in three sites. *Archives of General Psychiatry,* 41, 949-958.
17. Klerman, G. & Weissman, M. (1989). Increasing rates of Depression. *Journal of the American Medical Association,* 261, 2229-2235.

18. Klerman, G., Lavori, P., Rice, J., Reich, T., Endicott, J., Andreason, N., Keller, M., & Hirschfeld, R. (1985). Birth-cohort trends in rates of Major Depressive Disorder among relatives of patients with Affective Disorder. *Archives of General Psychiatry*, 42, 689-693.

19. Gutman, D.S. (2002). CME Medscape Psychiatry and Mental Health, Focus on Depression: Remission in Depression and the mind-body link. Retrieved July 5, 2003 from the World Wide Web: http://www.medscape.com/viewprogram/2067.

20. Cicchetti, D. (1991). A historical perspective on the discipline of developmental psychopathology. In J. Rolf, A.S. Masten, D. Cicchetti, K.H. Neuchterlein, & S. Weintraub (Eds). *Risk and Protective Factors in the Development of Psychopathology.* New York: Cambridge University Press.

21. Saudino, J.J., Pedersen, N.L., Lichenstein, P., McClearn, G.E., & Plomin, R. (1977). Can personality explain genetic influences on life events? *Journal of Personality and Social Psychology.* 72(1), 196-206.

22. Kendler, K.S., Kessler, R.C., Walters, E.E., MacLean, C., Neale, M.C., Heath, A.C., & Eaves, L.J. (1995). Stressful life events, genetic liability, and onset of an episode of major depression in women. *American Journal of Psychiatry*, 152, 833-842.

23. Suomi, S.J. (1999). Attachment in rhesus monkeys. In J. Cassidy & P. Shaver (Eds). *Handbook of Attachment: Theory, Research, and Clinical Applications,* New York: Guilford Press, (pp. 181-197).

24. Collins, W.A., Maccoby, E.E., Steinberg, L., Hetherington, E.M., & Bornstein, M.H. (2000). Contemporary research on parenting: The case for nature and nurture. *American Psychologist*, 55, 218-232.

25. Durand, V.M., & Barlow, D.H. (2003). *Essentials of Abnormal Psychology (3rd Ed.)*. Pacific Grove, CA: Thomson/Wadsworth.

26. Gutman, D., & Nemeroff, C.B. (2002). CME Medscape Psychiatry and Mental Health, Focus on Depression: The Neurobiology of Depression: Unmet Needs. Retrieved May, 2003 from the World Wide Web: http://www.medscape.com/viewprogram/2123_pnt.

27. Sadek, N., & Nemeroff, C. (2002). Update on the Neurobiology of Depression. CME Medscape: Psychiatry and Mental Health Treatment Updates. Retrieved October 17, 1999 from the World Wide Web: http://www.medscape.com/Medscape/psychiatry/TreatmentUpdate/2000/tu03/public/toc-tu03.html.

28. T. Joiner, & J.C. Coyne (1999). *Advances in Interpersonal Approaches: The Interactional Nature of Depression.* Washington, DC: American Psychological Association.

29. Holahan, C.J., Moos, R.H., & Bonin, L.A. (1999). Social context and depression: An integrative stress and coping framework. In T. Joiner & J.C. Coyne (Eds). *Advances in Interpersonal Approaches: The Interactional Nature of Depression,* (pp. 39-64). Washington, DC: American Psychological Association.

30. Stewart, J.R. (1998). Review of Beck Scale of Suicidal Ideation. In J.C. Impara & B.S. Plake (Eds). *The Thirteenth Mental Measurements Yearbook.* (Number 33, pp. 126-127) Lincoln, NE: Buros Institute.

31. Dill, J.C., & Anderson, C.A. (1999). Loneliness, shyness, and depression: The Etiology and interrelationships of everyday problems in living. In T. Joiner & J.C. Coyne (Eds). *Advances in Interpersonal Approaches: The Interactional Nature of Depression,* (pp. 93-126). Washington, DC: American Psychological Association.

32. Roberts, J.E., & Monroe, S.M. (1999). Vulnerable self-esteem and social process in depression: Toward an interpersonal model of self-esteem regulation. In T. Joiner & J.C. Coyne (Eds). *Advances in Interpersonal Approaches: The Interactional Nature of Depression,* (pp. 149-188). Washington, DC: American Psychological Association.

33. Sacco, W.P. (1999). A social-cognitive model of interpersonal processes in depression. In T. Joiner & J.C. Coyne (Eds). *Advances in Interpersonal Approaches: The Interactional Nature of Depression,* (pp. 329-362). Washington, DC: American Psychological Association.

34. Klinkman, M.S., Schwenk, T.L., & Coyne, J.C. (1997). Depression in primary care—More like asthma than appendicitis: The Michigan Depression Project. *Canadian Journal of Psychiatry,* 42, 966-973.

35. Sorenson, S.B., Rutter, C.M., & Aneshensel, C.S. (1991). Depression in the community: An investigation into age of onset. *Journal of Consulting and Clinical Psychology,* 59, 541-546.

36. Depression and Implications for Treatment. In S.R.H. Beach (Ed). *Marital and Family Processes in Depression: A Scientific Foundation for Clinical Practice.* Washington, DC: American Psychological Association.

37. Santor, D.A., Zuroff, D.C., Ramsay, P.C., & Palacios, J. (1995). Examining scale discriminability in the BDI and the CES-D as a function of depressive severity. *Psychological Assessment,* 7(2), 131-39.

38. Katz, R., Shaw, B.F., Vallis, T.M., Kaiser, A.S. (1995). The assessment of severity and symptom patterns in depression. In E.E. Beckham & W.R. Leber (Eds). *Handbook of Depression (2nd Ed),* New York: Guilford Press.

39. Carlson, J.F. (1998). Review of Beck Depression Inventory. In J.C. Impara & B.S. Plake (Eds). *The Thirteenth Mental Measurements Yearbook.* (Number 31, pp.117-119) Lincoln, NE: Buros Institute.

40. Ferketich, A.K., Schwartzbaum, J.A., Frid, D.J., & Moeschberger, M.L. (2000). Depression as an antecedent to heart disease among women and men in the NHANES I study. National Health and Nutrition Examination Survey. *Archives of Internal Medicine,* 160,1261-1268.

41. Broadley, A.J., Korszun, A., Jones, C.J., & Frenneaux, M.P. (2002). Arterial endothelial function is impaired in treated depression. *Heart,* 88, 521-523.

42. Joynt, K.E., Whellen, D.J., & O'Connor, C.M. (2003). Depression and cardiovascular disease: Mechanisms of interaction. *Biological Psychiatry,* 54(3), 248-261.

43. Beckham, E.E., Leber, W.R., & Youll, L.K. (1995). The diagnostic classification of depression. In E.E. Beckham & W.R. Leber (Eds). *Handbook of Depression (2nd Ed).* New York: Guildford Press.

44. Beck, A.T., Rush, A.J., Shaw, B.F., & Emery, G. (1979). *Cognitive Therapy of Depression.* New York: Guilford Press.

45. Bongar, B. (2002). *The Suicidal Patient: Clinical and Legal Standards of Care (2nd Ed).* Washington, DC: American Psychological Association.

46. Rudd, M.D., Joiner, T.E., Jobes, D.A., & King, C.A. (1999). The outpatient treatment of suicidality: An integration of science and recognition of its limitations. *Professional Psychology: Research and Practice,* 30(5), 437-446.

47. Stephens, D.E., Merikangas, K.R., & Merikangas, J.R. (1995). Comorbidity of depression and other medical conditions. In E.E. Beckham & W.R. Leber (Eds). *Handbook of Depression (2nd Ed).* New York: Guilford Press.

48. Kravitz, H.M., & Newman, A.J. (1995). Medical diagnostic procedures for depression: An update from a decade of promise. In E.E. Beckham & W.R. Leber (Eds). *Handbook of Depression (2nd Ed)*. New York: Guilford Press.

49. Koranyi, E. (1979). Morbidity and rate of undiagnosed physical illness in psychiatric clinic population. *Archives of General Psychiatry*, 36, 414-419.

50. Hall, R., Popkin, M., Devaul, R., Fallaice, L. & Stickney, S. (1978). Physical illness presenting as psychiatric disease. *Archives of General Psychiatry*, 35, 1315-1320.

51. National Institute of Mental Health. (2003). Suicide Facts. Downloaded June 28, 2003, from: http://www.nimh.nih.gov/research/suifact.cfm.

52. D. Hirschfeld, R.M., & Russell, J.M. (1997). Assessment and treatment of suicidal patients. *New England Journal of Medicine*. 333, 910-915.

53. E. Maris, R.W., Berman, A.L., & Silverman, M.M. (2000). *Comprehensive Textbook of Suicidology*. New York: Guilford Press.

54. Joiner, T.E., Walker, R.I., Rudd, M.D., Jobes, D.A. (1999). Scientizing and routinizing the assessment of suicidality in outpatient practice. Professional Psychology: *Research and Practice*, 30(5), 447-453.

55. Joiner, T.E., & Rudd, M.D. (2000). Intensity and duration of suicidal crises vary as a function of previous suicide attempts and negative life events. *Journal of Consulting and Clinical Psychology*, 68(5), 909-916.

56. Hasin, D.L., & Grant, B.F. (1987). Diagnosing depressive disorders in patients with alcohol and drug problems: A comparison of the SADS-L and the DIS. *Journal of Psychiatric Research*, 21(3), 301-311.

57. Maris, R.W. (1981). *Pathways to Suicide: A Survey of Self-destructive Behaviors*. Baltimore: John Hopkins University Press.

58. Maris, R.W., Berman, A.L., Matlsberger, J.T., & Yufit, R.I. (Eds) (1992). *Assessment and Prediction of Suicide*. New York, NY: Guilford Press.

59. Brink. T.L., Yesavage, J.A., Lum, O., et. al. (1982). Screening tests for geriatric depression. *Clinical Gerontologist*, 1(1), 37-43.

60. Murphy, L.L., Impara, J.C., Plake, B.S. (Eds). (1998) *Tests in Print V: An Index to Tests, Test Reviews, and the Literature on Specific Tests.* (Number 272, p.79) Lincoln, NE: Buros Institute.

61. Fernandez, E. (1998). Review of Beck Hopelessness Scale. In J.C. Impara & B.S. Plake (Eds). *The Thirteenth Mental Measurements Yearbook*. (Number 32, pp. 123-124). Lincoln, NE: Buros Institute.

62. Fernandez, E. (1998). Review of Beck Scale of Suicidal Ideation. In J.C. Impara & B.S. Plate (Eds). *The Thirteenth Mental Measurements Yearbook*. (Number 33, pp. 125-126). Lincoln, NE: Buros Institute.

63. Beck, A.T., Steer, R.A., & Ranieri, W.F. (1988). Scale for suicide ideation: Psychometric properties of a self-report version. *Journal of Clinical Psychology*, 44, 500-505.

64. Beck, A.T., Kovacs, M. & Weissman, A. (1979). Assessment of suicidal intention: The scale for suicide ideation. *Journal of Consulting and Clinical Psychology*, 47, 343-352.

65. Golding, S.L. (1985). Review of Suicide Probability Scale. In J.V. Mitchell, Jr. (Ed). *The Ninth Mental Measurements Yearbook, Vol. II.* Lincoln, NE: Buros Institute.

66. Farbernow, N.L., Helig, S. & Litman, R. (1968). *Techniques in Crisis Intervention: A Training Manual*. Los Angeles: Suicide Prevention Center.

67. Reynolds, W.M. (1991). *Adult Suicidal Ideation Questionnaire: Professional Manual*. Odessa, FL: Psychological Assessment Resources.

68. Reynolds, W.M. & Mazza, J.J. (1992). *Suicidal Behavior History Form: Clinician's Guide*. Odessa, FL: Psychological Assessment Resources.

69. Weissman, A.D., & Worden, J.W. (1974). Risk-rescue in suicide assessment. *Archives of General Psychiatry*, 26, 553-560.

70. Smith, K., Conroy, R.W., & Ehler, B.D. (1984). Lethality of suicide attempt rating scale. *Suicide & Life Threatening Behavior*, 14(4), 215-242.

71. Linehand, M.M. (1985). The reasons for living inventory. In P. Keller & L. Ritt (Eds). *Innovations in Clinical Practice,* (pp. 321-330). Sarasota, FL: Professional Resource Exchange.

72. Brody, D.S., Hahn, S.R., Spitzer, R.L., Kroenke, K., Linzer, M., deGriy, F.V., & Williams, J.B. (1998). Identifying patients with depression in primary care settings: A more efficient method. *Archives of Internal Medicine*, 158, 2469-2475.

73. Richards, K., & Range, L.M. (2001). Is training in psychology associated with increased responsiveness to suicidality? *Death Studies*, 25, 265-279.

74. Buelow, G., & Range, L.M. (2001). No-suicide contracts among college students. *Death Studies*, 25, 583-592.

75. Rudd, M.D., Joiner, T.E., Jobes, D.A., King, C.A. (1999). The outpatient treatment of suicidality: An integration of science and recognition of its limitations. *Professional Psychology: Research and Practice*, 30(5), 437-446.

76. Beutler, L.E. (2000). David and Goliath: When empirical and clinical standards of practice meet. *American Psychologist*, 55(9), 997-1007.

77. Andrews-Clarke v. Travelers, 984 F Supp. 49 (1997).

78. White, T.W. (2003). Legal issues and suicide risk management. *The National Psychologist*, 12(2), 12.

79. Norcross, J.C., Hedges, M., Castle, P.H. (2002). Psychologists conducting psychotherapy in 2001: A study of the Division 29 membership. *Psychotherapy: Theory/Research/Practice/Training*, 39(1), 97-102.

80. Getz, M., Pedersen, W.S., Plomin, R., Messelroade, J.R., and McClearn, G.E., (1992). Importance of shared genes and shared environments for symptoms of Depression in older adults. *Archives of General Psychiatry*, 101, 701-708.

81. Blatt, S.J. (1974). Levels of object representation in anaclitic and introjective Depression. *The Psychoanalytic Study of the Child*, 29, 107-57.

82. Shapiro, D.A., Barkham, M., Rees, A., Hardy, G.E., Reynolds, S., & Startup, M. (1994). Effects of treatment duration and severity of depression on the effectiveness of cognitive-behavioral and psychodynamic-interpersonal psychotherapy. *Journal of Consulting and Clinical Psychology*, 62, 522-534.

83. Shapiro, D.A., & Firth, J.A. (1987). Prescriptive vs. exploratory psychotherapy: outcomes of the Sheffield Psychotherapy Project. *British Journal of Psychiatry*, 151, 790-799.

84. Reck, C., & Mundt, C. (2002). Psychodynamic therapy approaches in depressive disorders. Pathogenesis models and empirical principles. [Original in German]. *Nervenarzt*, 73(7), 613-619.

85. Eysenck, H.C. (1993). Psychoanalysis: Pseudo-science. (Letter to the editor), *American Psychological Association Monitor*, 24 (8) p. 4.

86. McLean, P.D. & Hakstian, A.R. (1979). Clinical depression: Comparative efficacy of outpatient treatments. *Journal of Consulting and Clinical Psychology*, 47, 818-836.

87. Giles, T.R. (1993). *Handbook of Effective Psychotherapy,* New York: Plenum Press.

88. Rachman, S.J., & Wilson, G.T. (1980). *The Effects of Psychotherapy (2nd ed.)*. New York: Pergamon Press.

89. Karau, T.B., Gelenberg, A., Merriam, A., & Wang, P. (2000). Practice guidelines for the treatment of patients with major depressive disorder (Revision). *American Journal of Psychiatry*, 157(4), (April 2000 Supplement).

90. Nathan, P.E. & Gorman, J.M. (Eds). (1998). *A Guide to Treatments that Work*. New York: Oxford University Press.

91. Gabbard, G.O., Gunderson, J.G., Fonagy, P. (2002). The place of psychoanalytic treatments within psychiatry. *Archives of General Psychiatry*, 59(6), 505-510.

92. Burnand, Y., Andreoli, A., Kolatte, E., Venturini, A., & Rossen, N. (2002). Psychodynamic psychotherapy and climipramine in the treatment of major depression. *Psychiatric Services*, 53(5), 585-590.

93. Barkham, M., Shapiro, D.A., Hardy, G.E., Rees, A. (1999). Psychotherapy in two-plus-one sessions: outcomes of a randomized controlled trial of Cognitive-Behavioral and Psychodynamic-Interpersonal therapy for subsyndromal depression. *Journal of Consulting and Clinical Psychology*, 67(2), 201-211.

94. Elkin, I., Shea, T., Watkins, J.T., Imber, S.D., Sotsky, S.M., Collins, J.F., Glass, D.R., Pilkonis, P.A., Leber, W.R., Docherty, J.P., Giester, S.J., Parloff, J.B. (1989). National Institute of Mental Health treatment of Depression collaborative research program: General effectiveness of treatments. *Archives of General Psychiatry*, 46, 971-982.

95. Craighead, W.E., Craighead, L.W., & Ilardi, S.S., (1998). Psychosocial treatments for Major Depressive Disorder. In P.E. Nathan & J.M. Gorman (Eds). *A Guide to Treatments that Work*. New York: Oxford University Press.

96. Klerman, G., Weissman, M., Rounsaville, B., & Chevron, E. (1984) *Interpersonal Psychotherapy of Depression*, New York: Basic Books.

97. Klerman, G. & Weissman, M. (1993). Interpersonal psychotherapy for depression: Background and concepts. In G.L. Klerman and M.M. Weissman (Eds). *New applications of interpersonal psychotherapy.* Washington, DC: American Psychiatric Press.

98. Weissman, M.M., Klerman, G.L., Prusoff, B.A., Sholomskas, D., & Padian, N. (1981). Depressed outpatients: Results one year after treatment with drugs and/or interpersonal psychotherapy. *Archives of General Psychiatry*, 38, 51-55.

99. Weissman, M.M., Prusoff, B.A., DiMascio, A., Neu, Glokaney, & Klerman, G.L. (1979) The efficacy of drugs and psychotherapy in the treatment of acute depressive episodes. *American Journal of Psychiatry*, 136, 555-558.

100. Lewinsohn, P.M., Sullivan, J.M., & Grosscup, S.J. (1980). Changing reinforcing events: An approach to the treatment of depression. *Psychotherapy: Theory, Research, and Practice*, 47. 322-334.

101. Jacobson, N.S., Dobson, K.S., Truax, P.A., Addis, M.E., Koerner, K., Gollan, J.K., Gortner, E. & Prince, S.E. (1996). A component analysis of cognitive-behavioral treatment for depression. *Journal of Consulting and Clinical Psychology*, 64, 74-80.

102. Yankura, J., and Dryden, W. (1990). *Doing RET: Albert Ellis in Action.* New York: Springer Publishing.

103. Ellis, A. (1976). The Biological basis of human irrationality. *Journal of Individual Psychology.* 32, 145-168.

104. Beck, A.T., Rush, A.J., Shaw, B.F., & Emery, G. (1979). *Cognitive Therapy of Depression.* New York: Guilford Press.

105. Beck, A.T., & Freeman, A. (1990). *Cognitive Therapy of Personality Disorders.* New York: Guilford Press.

106. Robins, C.J., & Hayes, A.M. (1993). An appraisal of cognitive therapy. *Journal of Consulting and Clinical Psychology,* 61, 205-214.

107. Smith, M.L., & Glass, G.V. (1977). Meta-analysis of psychotherapy outcome studies. *American Psychologist,* 32, 752-760.

108. Lyons, L.C., Woods, P.J. (1991). The efficacy of rational-emotive therapy: A quantitative review of the outcome research. *Clinical Psychology Review,* 11, 357-369.

109. Hollon, S.D., Shelton, R.C., & Loosen, P.T. (1991). Cognitive therapy and pharmacotherapy for depression. *Journal of Consulting and Clinical Psychology,* 59, 88-99.

110. Beck. A.T. (1993). Cognitive therapy: Past, present, and future. *Journal of Consulting and Clinical Psychology,* 61, 194-198.

111. Scott, J., Palmer, S., Paykel, E., Teasdale, J., & Hayhurst, H. (2003). Use of cognitive therapy for relapse prevention in chronic depression: A cost-effective study. *British Journal of Psychiatry,* 182, 221-227.

112. Shaw, B.F. (1977). Comparison of cognitive therapy and behavior therapy in the treatment of depression. *Journal of Consulting and Clinical Psychology,* 45, 543-551.

113. Gioe, V.J. (1975). Cognitive modification and positive group experience as a treatment for depression. Doctoral dissertation, Temple University. *Dissertation Abstracts International,* 36, 3039B-3040B (University microfilms 75-28, 219.)

114. Covi, L., Roth, D., & Lipman, R.S. (1982). Cognitive group psychotherapy of depression: The close-ended group. *American Journal of Psychotherapy,* 36, 459-460.

115. Yalom, I.D. (1975). *The Theory and Practice of Group Psychotherapy (2nd Ed.).* New York: Basic Books.

116. Yalom, I.D. (1983). *Inpatient Group Psychotherapy.* New York: Basic Books.

117. Lewinsohn, P.M., Antonuccio, D.O., Breckenridge, J., & Jeri, L. (1984). *The Coping with Depression Course: A Psychoeducational Interview for Unipolar Depression.* Eugene, OR: Castalia Publishing Co.

118. Luby, J.L., & Yalom, I.D. (1992). Group therapy. In E.S. Paykel (Ed). (1992). *Handbook of Affective Disorders (2nd Ed.).* New York: Guilford Press.

119. Clarke, G., & Lewinsohn, P.M. (1989). The Coping with Depression Course: A group psychoeducational intervention for unipolar Depression. *Behavior Change,* 6, 54-69.

120. Kohn, L.P., Oden, T., Munoz, R.F., Robinson, A., Leavitt, D. (2002). Adapted cognitive behavioral group therapy for depressed low-income African American women. *Community Mental Health Journal,* 38(6), 497-504.

121. Beach, S.R.H. (2001). Marital therapy for co-occurring marital discord and depression. In S.R.H. Beach (Ed). *Marital and Family Processes in Depression: A Scientific Foundation for Clinical Practice.* Washington, DC: American Psychological Association.

122. Gotlib, I.H., & McCabe, S.B. (1990). Marriage and Psychopathology. In F.D. Fincham & T.N. Bradbury (Eds.). *The Psychology of Marriage: Basic Issues and Applications.* New York: Guilford Press.

123. Paykel, E.S., Myers, J.K., Dienelt, M.N., Klerman, G.L., Lindenthal, J.J., &Pepper, M.P. (1969). Life events and depression: A controlled study. *Archives of General Psychiatry*, 21, 753-760.

124. Vaughn, C.E., & Leff, J.P. (1976). The influence of family and social factors on the course of psychiatric illness: A comparison of schizophrenic and depressed neurotic patients. *British Journal of Psychiatry*, 129, 125-137.

125. Merikangas, K.R. (1982). Divorce and assortative mating for psychiatric disorders and psychological traits. *Archives of General Psychiatry*, 141, 74-76.

126. Costello, C.G. (1982). Social factors associated with depression: A retrospective community study. *Psychological Medicine*, 12, 329-339.

127. Prince, S.E. & Jacobson, N.S. (1995). Couple and family therapy for depression. In E.E. Beckham & W.R. Leber (Eds). *Handbook of Depression (2nd Ed).* New York: Guilford Press.

128. Beutler, L.E., Clarkin, J.F., & Bonger, B. (2000). *Guidelines for the Systematic Treatment of the Depressed Patient.* New York. Oxford University Press.

129. Carey, G. & Dilalla, D.L. (1994). Personality and psychopathology: Genetic perspective. *Journal of Abnormal Psychology*, 103, 32-43.

130. Miller, I.W., Norman, W.H., & Keitner, G.I. (1990). Treatment response of high cognitive dysfunction depressed inpatients. *Comprehensive Psychiatry*, 30, 61-72.

131. Lickey, M.E. & Gordon, B. (1983). *Drugs for Mental Illness: A Revolution in Psychiatry.* New York: W H. Freeman and Co.

132. Kolb, B. & Whishaw, I. (1985). *Fundamentals of Human Neuropsychology (2nd Ed.).* New York, NY: W.H. Freeman and Co.

133. Gutman, D., & Nemeroff, C.B. (2002). CME Medscape Psychiatry and Mental Health, Focus on Depression: The Neurobiology of Depression: Unmet Needs. Retrieved May, 2003 from the World Wide Web: http://www.medscape.com/viewprogram/2123_pnt.

134. Sammons, M.T. (2001). Combined Treatments for Mental Disorders: Clinical Dilemmas. In Sammons, M.T., & Schmidt, N.B. (Eds). *Combined Treatments for Mental Disorders: A Guide to Psychological and Pharmacological Interventions.* Washington, DC: American Psychological Association.

135. Goldberg, J.F., & Whiteside, S.E. (2002). The association between substance abuse and antidepressant-induced mania: A preliminary study. *Journal of Clinical Psychiatry*, 63(9), 791-795

136. Egli, D. (2002). CE American Psychological Association, Division 55: If An SSRI, Which One First? Retrieved May 25, 2003 from the World Wide Web at: http://www.apa.org/divisions/div55/CE/EgliOnSSRIs.htm.

137. Nemeroff, C.B. & Schatzberg, A.F. (1998). Pharmacological Treatment of Unipolar Depression. In P.E. Nathan & J.M. Gorman (Eds). *A Guide to Treatments that Work.* New York: Oxford University Press.

138. Preskorn, S.H. (1999). *Outpatient Management of Depression: A Guide for the Practitioner, 2nd Edition*. Professional Communications: Caddo, Oklahoma.

139. Quitkin, F.M., Stewart, J.W., McGrath, P.J., Taylor, B.P., Tisminetzky, M.S., Petkova, E., Chen, Y., Ma, G., & Klein, D.F. (2002). Are there differences between women and men's antidepressant responses? *American Journal of Psychiatry*, 159, 1848-1854.

140. Thase, M.E. & Kupfer, D.J. (1996). Recent developments in the pharmacotherapy of mood disorders. *Journal of Consulting and Clinical Psychology*, 64, 646-659.

141. Preston, J., & Ebert, B. (1999). Psychologists' role in the discussion of psychotropic medication with clients: Legal and ethical considerations. *California Psychologist*, October, 32, 34.

142. Barclay, L. (2004). Algorithm-Based Program Effective for Major Depressive Disorder. CME Medscape: Medical News (CME Author: Lie, D.). Retrieved July 20, 2004 from the World Wide Web: http://www.medscape.com/viewarticle/482774?SRC=mp.

143. Crismon, M.L., Trivedi, M., Pigott, T.A., Rushe, A. J., Hirschfeld, R.M., Kahn, D.A., DeBattista, Cl, Nelson, J.C., Nierenberg, A.A., Sackeim, H.A., Thase, M.E. (1999). The Texas Medication Algorithm Project: report of the Texas Consensus Conference Panel on Medication Treatment of Major Depressive Disorder. *J Clin Psychiatry*. Mar;60(3):142-56.

144. Texas Department of State Health Services. Texas Implementation of Medication Algorithms (Depression Algorithm). Retrieved December 22, 2004 from the World Wide Web: http://www.dshs.state.tx.us/mhprograms/TIMA.shtm.

145. Keller, M.B. & Boland, R.J. (1998). Implications of failing to achieve successful long-term maintenance treatment of recurrent unipolar major depression. *Biological Psychiatry*, 44, 348-360.

146. Akiskal, H.S. (1985). The clinical management of affective disorders. In R. Michels, J.O. Cavenar, K.H. Brodie, A.M. Cooper, S.B. Guze, L.L. Judd, G.L. Klerman, and A.J. Soinit (eds.), *Psychiatry*, 1, 1-27. Philadelphia: Lippincott.

147. Bortman, A.W., Falk, W.E., and Gelberg, A.J. (1987). Pharmacologic treatment of acute depressive subtypes. In H.Y. Meltzer (Ed.), *Psychopharmacology: The Third Generation of Progress,* (pp. 1031-1040). New York: Raven Press.

148. Frangos, E., Tsitourides, A.S., Psilolignos, P., and Katsanou, N. (1983). Psychotic depressive disorder: A separate entity? *Journal of Affective Disorders*, 5, 259-265.

149. Antonuccio, D.O. (1993). Psychotherapy vs. medication for depression: Challenging the conventional wisdom. Paper presented at the annual meeting of the American Psychological Association. Toronto, Canada.

150. U.S. Food and Drug Administration (2004). FDA Talk Paper: FDA Issues Public Health Advisory on Cautions for Use of Antidepressants in Adults and Children (T04-08, March 22, 2004). Downloaded from: http://www.fda.gov.

151. Conte, H.R., Plutchik, R., Wild, K.V., & Karasu, T.B. (1986). Combined psychotherapy and pharmacotherapy for depression: A systematic analysis of the evidence. *Archives of General Psychiatry*, 43, 471-479.

152. Pettit, J.W., Voelz, Z.R., & Joiner, T.E. (2001). Combined treatments for depression. In Sammons, M.T., & Schmidt, N.B. (Eds). *Combined Treatments for Mental Disorders: A Guide to Psychological and Pharmacological Interventions.* Washington, DC: American Psychological Association.

153. Keller, M.B., McCullough, J.P., Klein, D.N., Arnow, B., Dunner, D.L., Gelenberg, A.J., Markowitz, J.C., Nemeroff, C.B., Russel, J.M., Thase, M.E., Trivedi, M.H., & Zajecka, J. (2000). A comparison of nefazadone, the cognitive behavioral analysis system of psychotherapy and their conbination for the treatment of chronic depression. *New England Journal of Medicine*, 342, 1462-1470.

154. Albers, L.J., Kahn, R.K., & Reist, C. (2001). *Handbook of Psychiatric Drugs*, Laguna Hills, CA: Current Clinical Strategies Publishing.

155. Weiner, R.D. (1979). The psychiatric use of electrically induced seizures. *American Journal of Psychiatry, 131*, 1507-1517.

156. Turek, I.S., & Hanlon, T.P. (1977). The effectiveness and safety of electroconvulsive therapy (ECT). *Journal of Nervous and Mental Disease*, 164, 419-431.

157. Fink, M. (1978). Efficacy and safety of induced seizure (EST) in man. *Comprehensive Psychiatry*, 19, 1-18.

158. Fink, M. (1992). Electroconvulsive therapy. In E.S. Paykel (Ed.). *Handbook of Affective Disorders (2nd Ed.)*. New York: Guilford Press.

159. Avery, D. & Lubrano, A. (1979). Depression treated with imipramine and ECT: The DeCarolis study reconsidered. *American Journal of Psychiatry*, 136, 559-562.

160. Philipp M, Kohnen R, & Hiller KO. (1999) Hypericum extract versus imipramine or placebo in patients with moderate depression: Randomized multicentre study of treatment for eight weeks. *BMJ*, 319, 1534-1538.

161. Laakmann G, Schule C, Baghai T, et. al. (1998). St. John's wort in mild to moderate depression: the Relevance of hyperforin for the clinical efficacy. *Pharmacopsychiatry*, 31(Supplement 1), 54-59.

162. Kim, H.L., Streltzer, J., & Goebert, D. (1999). St. John's Wort for depression: A Metaanalysis of well defined clinical trials. *Journal of Nervous and Mental Diseases*, 187(9), 532-538.

163. Linde K., Mulrow, CD. (2004) St John's wort for depression (Cochrane Review). In: *The Cochrane Library*, Issue 4. Chichester, UK: John Wiley & Sons, Ltd.

164. Chen, J.J. (2002). An Evidence-based Assessment of Glucosamine Sulfate, St. John's Wort, and Echinacea. Based on proceedings from the 36th Annual Mid-year Conference of the American Society of Health-System Pharmacists, New Orleans, LA, December 2-6, 2001.

165. Tkachuk, G.A. & Martin, G.L. (1999). Exercise therapy for patients with psychiatric disorders: Research and clinical implications. *Professional Psychology: Research and Practice*. 30, 275-282..

166. Gutman, A.R., Gutman, D., Nemeroff, C.B. (2002). CME Medscape Psychiatry and Mental Health, Focus on Depression: New Vistas in Antidepressant Development. Retrieved May, 2003 from http://www.medscape.com/viewprogram/2131_pnt.

167. DeVane, C.L. (2001). Substance P: A new era, a new role. *Pharmacotherapy*, 21(9), 1061-1069.

168. Haddjeri, N. & Blier, P. (2001). Sustained blockade of neurokinin-1 receptors enhances serotonin neurotransmission. *Biological Psychiatry*, 50(3), 191-199

169. Bilkei-Gorzo, A., Racz, I., Michel, K., & Zimmer, A. (2002). Diminished anxiety- and depression- related behaviors in mice with selective destruction of the tac1 gene. *Journal of Neuroscience*, 22(22), 10046-10052

170. Martin, J.L.R., Barbanoj, M.J., Schlaepfer, T.E., Clos, S., et. al. (2003). Transcranial magnetic stimulation for treating depression. *Cochrane Database of Systematic Reviews (vol. 3)*. Online at www.cochrane.org.

171. Bender, K.J. (2002), EEG predicts antidepressant responders. *Psychiatric Times (Advances in Psychiatric Medicine)*, 19(8), 9.

172. Zung, W. (1965). A self-rating depression scale. *Archives of General Psychiatry*, 12, 63-70.

173. Radloff, L. (1977). The CES-D scale: A self-report depression scale for research in the general population. *Applied Psychological Measurement*, 1, 385-401.

174. Beck, A., Ward, C., Mendelson, J., Mack, J. & Erbaugh, J. (1961). An inventory for measuring depression. *Archives of General Psychiatry*, 4, 561-571.

175. Coyne, J. (1994). Self-reported distress: Analog or ersatz Depression? *Psychological Bulletin*. 116 (1). 29-45.

176. Fechner-Bates, S., Coyne, J., & Schwenk, T. (1994). The relationship of self-reported distress to depressive disorders and other psychopathology. *Journal of Consulting and Clinical Psychology*, 62, 550-559.

177. Steer, R.A., Beck, A.T., Clark, D.A. & Beck, J.S. (1994). Psychometric properties of the Cognition Checklist with psychiatric outpatients and university students. *Psychological Assessment*, 6(1), 67-70.

178. Clark, D.A.; Cook, A., & Snow, D. (1998). Depressive symptom differences in hospitalized, medically ill, depressed psychiatric inpatients and nonmedical controls. *Journal of Abnormal Psychology*, 107(1), 38-48.

179. Holroyd, S., & Clayton, A.H. (2000). Measuring Depression in the Elderly: Which scale is best? *Medscape Mental Health*, 5(5). Retrieved September 26, 2000 from the World Wide Web: http://psychiatry.medscape.com/Medscape/psychiatry/journal/2000/v05.n05/mh3033.holr

180. Alexopoulous, G.S., Abrams, R.C., Young, R.C., & Shamoian, C.A. (1988). Cornell Scale for Depression in Dementia. *Biological Psychiatry*, 23(3), 271-284.

181. Hamilton, M. (1960). A rating scale for depression. *Journal of Neurology and Neurosurgical Psychiatry*, 12, 56-62.

182. Brown, C., Schulberg, H.C., Madonia, M.J. (1995). Assessment depression in primary care practice with the Beck Depression Inventory and the Hamilton Rating Scale for Depression. *Psychological Assessment*, 7(1), 59-65.

183. Kobak, K.A., Reynolds, W.M., Rosenfeld, R. & Greist, J.H. (1990). Development and validation of a computer-administered version of the Hamilton Depression Rating Scale. *Psychological Assessment*, 2(1), 56-63.

184. Reynolds, W.M., Kobak, K.A. (1995). Reliability and validity of the Hamilton Depression Inventory: A paper-and-pencil version of the Hamilton Depression Rating Scale Clinical Interview. *Psychological Assessment*, 7(4), 472-483.

185. First, M., Spitzer, L., Gibbon, M. & Williams, J. (1995). *Structured Clinical Interview for Axis I DSM-IV Disorders (SCID Version 2.0)*. Washington, DC: American Psychiatric Press.

186. Endicott, J. (1986). Schedule for Affective Disorders and Schizophrenia, Regular and Change versions: Measure of depression. In N. Sartorius & T.A. Ban (Eds). *Assessment of Depression*. Heidelberg: Springer-Verlag.

187. Robins, L.N., Cottler, L., Bucholz, K. (1995). *Diagnostic Interview Schedule for DSM-IV*. St. Louis: Washington University.

188. Blouin, A.G., Perez, E.L., & Blouin, J.H. (1988). Computerized administration of the Diagnostic Interview Schedule. *Psychiatry Research*, 22 (3), 335-344.

189. Robins, L.N., Wing, J., Wittchen, H.U., Helzer, J.E., Babor, T.F., Burke, J., Farmer, A., Jablenski, A.,Pickens, R., Regier, D.A., Sartorius, N. & Towle, L.H. (1988). The Composite International Diagnostic Interview: An epidemiologic instrument suitable for use in conjunction with different diagnostic systems and in different cultures. *Archives of General Psychiatry*, 45, 1069-1077.

190. World Health Organization (1997). *Composite International Diagnostic Interview Schedule for DSM-IV, Version 2.1*, Geneva: World Health Organization.

191. Whooley, M.A., Avins, A.I., Miranda, J. & Browner, W.S. (1997). Case-finding instruments for depression: Two questions are as good as many. *Journal of General Internal Medicine*, 12, 439-445.

192. Spitzer, R.L., Kroenke, K., & Williams, J.B. (1999). Validation and utility of the self-report version of the PRIME-MD: The Primary Care Study. *Journal of the American Medical Association*, 282, 1737.

193. Baer, L., Jacobs, D.G., Meszler-Reizes, J., Blais, M., Fava, M., Kessler, R., Magruder, K., Murphy, J., Kopans, B., Cukor, P., Leahy, L., O'Laughlen, J. (2000). Development of a brief screening instrument: The HANDS. *Psychotherapy and Psychosomatics*, 69(1), 35-41.

194. Beck, A.T., Brown, G.K., Steer, R.A., Dahlsgaard, K.K., & Grisham, J.R. (1999). Suicide ideation at its worst point: A predictor of eventual suicide in psychiatric outpatients. *Suicide & Life Threatening Behavior*, 29(1), 1-9.

195. Exner, J.E. (1993). *The Rorschach: A Comprehensive System: Volume 1: Basic Foundations*, Somerset, New Jersey: John Wiley and Sons.

196. Hathaway, S.R., & McKinley, J.C. (1983). *The Minnesota Multiphasic Personality Inventory Manual*. New York: Psychological Corporation.

197. Hathaway, S.R., Butcher, J.N., & McKinley, J.C. (1989). *Minnesota Multiphasic Personality Inventory - 2*, Minneapolis, MN: University of Minnesota Press.

198. Graham, J.R. (1990). *MMPI-2: Assessing Personality and Psychopathology*, New York: Oxford University Press.

Index

N

P

R

S

T

V

W

Y

Z

We Want Your Opinion!

Comments about **Depression in Adults**:

____

____

____

____

____

Other titles you would like Compact Clinicals to offer:

____

____

____

____

To be placed on our mailing list, please provide the following:

Name: ______________________________

Address: ______________________________

____

____

E-mail: ______________________________

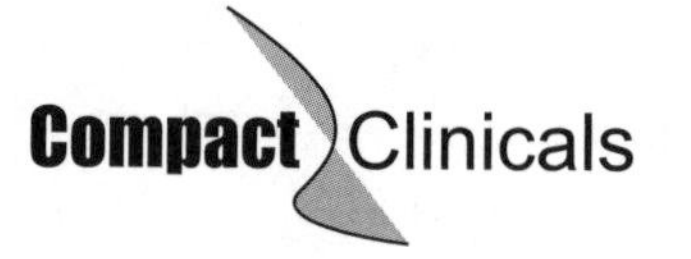

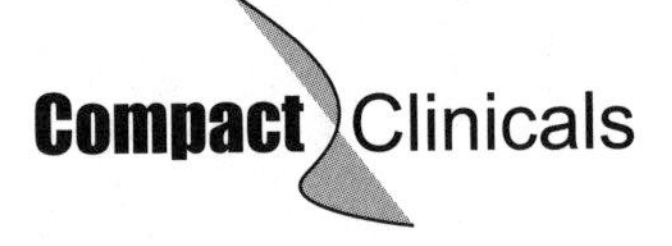

Order in 3 easy steps:

▶ 1 Provide complete billing and shipping information

Name ______________________ Company ______________________

Profession ______________________ Dept./Mail Stop ______________________

Street Address/P.O. Box ______________________

City/State/Zip ______________________

Telephone ______________________ ☐ Ship to Residence ☐ Ship to Business

▶ 2 Choose Titles

Title	Qty.	Unit Price	Total
Attention Deficit Hyperactivity Disorder *The latest assessment and treatment strategies*		$16.95	
Bipolar Disorder *The latest assessment and treatment strategies*		$16.95	
Bipolar Disorder: Treatment and Management		$18.95	
Borderline Personality Disorder *The latest assessment and treatment strategies*		$16.95	
Conduct Disorders *The latest assessment and treatment strategies*		$16.95	
Depression in Adults *The latest assessment and treatment strategies*		$16.95	
Obsessive Compulsive Disorder *The latest assessment and treatment strategies*		$16.95	
Post Traumatic Stress Disorder *The latest assessment and treatment strategies*		$16.95	
		Subtotal	
		Tax (Add 7.975% in MO)	
		Shipping ($3.75 first book/ $1.00 per additional book)	
		TOTAL	

Continuing Education credits available for mental health professionals. Call 1-800-408-8830 for details.

▶ 3 Choose Payment Method

Please charge my: ☐ Visa ☐ MasterCard ☐ Discover ☐ American Express ☐ Check Enclosed

Account # ____ – ____ – ____ – ____ Exp. Date ___/___

Name on Card ______________________ Cardholder Signature ______________________

Postal Orders: Compact Clinicals, 7205 NW Waukomis Dr., Suite A, Kansas City, MO 64151

We Want Your Opinion!

Comments about **Depression in Adults**:

____

____

____

____

____

Other titles you would like Compact Clinicals to offer:

____

____

____

____

To be placed on our mailing list, please provide the following:

Name: ____

Address: ____

____

____

E-mail: ____

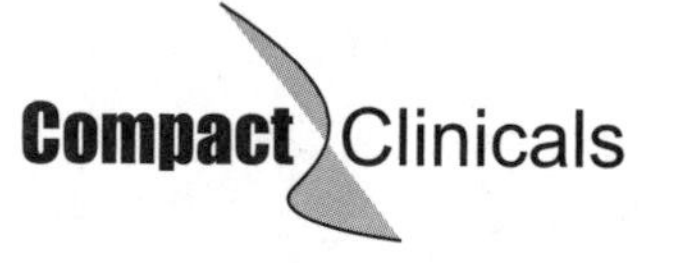

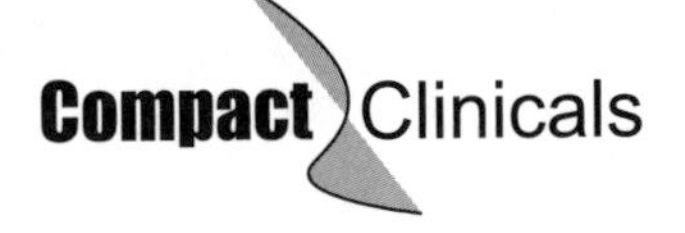

Order in 3 easy steps:

▶ 1 Provide complete billing and shipping information

Name ______________________ Company ______________________

Profession ______________________ Dept./Mail Stop ______________________

Street Address/P.O. Box ______________________

City/State/Zip ______________________

Telephone ______________________ ☐ Ship to Residence ☐ Ship to Business

▶ 2 Choose Titles

	Qty.	Unit Price	Total
Attention Deficit Hyperactivity Disorder *The latest assessment and treatment strategies*		$16.95	
Bipolar Disorder *The latest assessment and treatment strategies*		$16.95	
Bipolar Disorder: Treatment and Management		$18.95	
Borderline Personality Disorder *The latest assessment and treatment strategies*		$16.95	
Conduct Disorders *The latest assessment and treatment strategies*		$16.95	
Depression in Adults *The latest assessment and treatment strategies*		$16.95	
Obsessive Compulsive Disorder *The latest assessment and treatment strategies*		$16.95	
Post Traumatic Stress Disorder *The latest assessment and treatment strategies*		$16.95	
		Subtotal	
		Tax (Add 7.975% in MO)	
		Shipping ($3.75 first book/ $1.00 per additional book)	
		TOTAL	

Continuing Education credits available for mental health professionals. Call 1-800-408-8830 for details.

▶ 3 Choose Payment Method

Please charge my: ☐ Visa ☐ MasterCard ☐ Discover ☐ American Express ☐ Check Enclosed

Account # ____ – ____ – ____ – ____ Exp. Date __ __ / __ __

Name on Card ______________________ Cardholder Signature ______________________

Postal Orders: Compact Clinicals, 7205 NW Waukomis Dr., Suite A, Kansas City, MO 64151